# Increase
# Your
# HEIGHT

# Increase Your HEIGHT

(You will read in this book about the well tried devices and revolutionary principles involved in increasing your height in a natural way. These are based on researches yielding wonderful results. With the help of these devices and principles, you can succeed in increasing your height to your heart's desire.)

Krishna Gopal Vikal

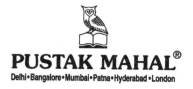

**PUSTAK MAHAL®**
Delhi•Bangalore•Mumbai•Patna•Hyderabad•London

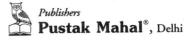

*Publishers*
## Pustak Mahal®, Delhi

J-3/16 , Daryaganj, New Delhi-110002
☎ 23276539, 23272783, 23272784 • *Fax:* 011-23260518
*E-mail:* info@pustakmahal.com • *Website:* www.pustakmahal.com

**London Office**
5, Roddell Court, Bath Road, Slough SL3 OQJ, England
*E-mail:* pustakmahaluk@pustakmahal.com

**Sales Centre**
10-B, Netaji Subhash Marg, Daryaganj, New Delhi-110002
☎ 23268292, 23268293, 23279900 • *Fax:* 011-23280567
*E-mail:* rapidexdelhi@indiatimes.com

**Branch Offices**
**Bangalore:** ☎ 22234025
*E-mail:* pmblr@sancharnet.in • pustak@sancharnet.in
**Mumbai:** ☎ 22010941
*E-mail:* rapidex@bom5.vsnl.net.in
**Patna:** ☎ 3294193 • *Telefax:* 0612-2302719
*E-mail:* rapidexptn@rediffmail.com
**Hyderabad:** *Telefax:* 040-24737290
*E-mail:* pustakmahalhyd@yahoo.co.in

© **Pustak Mahal, Delhi**

ISBN 978-81-223-0093-2

**Edition : 2007**

*Printed at :* Unique Colour Carton, Mayapuri, Delhi-110064

# Preface

You will find in this book the well tried devices to increase your height. These are equally applicable to men as well as women. The techniques outlined here are the result of serious and prolonged researches. The fundamental principles arrived at are quite revolutionary in nature.

The very great popularity enjoyed by the book, which was originally published in Hindi, has encouraged us to bring out an English version of the book for the benefit of those readers, who prefer to read in English language.

It is no doubt a fact that our stature very much depends upon our heredity, but it is equally true to say that if we pay attention from the very beginning and make efforts, the height of the offspring can be increased by gradually eliminating those factors which check the growth of stature from one generation to another.

A tall stature has its definite and positive role to play in the development of an effective personality. There is no doubt that a person who is not tall cannot enjoy his life as happier as a tall person can. Tall persons are usually preferred in the services of police, military and big companies. If you want to select a bride for your son, you will normally prefer a girl who is tall. Similarly girls like tall boys as their partners in life. These examples go to show that a short-statured person often lags behind in the actual race of life.

We want to assure you that, through the medium of this book we have tried to achieve the impossible. For the first time in India this Course has been published which is fully illustrated. It has already been successfully practised in England and America. If you will practise Courses given in the book for fifteen minutes per day with faith and self-confidence, you can increase your height by 4 to 10 cm within a few weeks.

It is the speciality of this Course that by practising it regularly with full faith and confidence, the height of a person does not increase by his legs alone, but the length of the backbone also increases gradually. In Part Four of the book, you will find the solution of a number of problems which arise in your mind while practising the Course. We have also given some well-tried Dieting Charts towards the end of the book for your guidance.

We have every hope that the book will prove a boon to persons of all ages. Think high, climb high and 'Go Ahead'! Our best wishes are with you.

—PUBLISHERS

# Contents

| | |
|---|---|
| **PART ONE: THE PROBLEM** | **9-17** |

Short stature: A curse—Short stature: An all pervading problem—Stature and our point of view—The opinion of doctors and our programme entitled "Increase Your Height and Improve Your Posture"—The basis of our programme —How can height be reduced or increased?—What is the significance of 'Adequate Height'?—What is an ideal height? —How to establish an ideal symmetry between the various parts of our body?

| | |
|---|---|
| **PART TWO: THE KNOWLEDGE** | **19-68** |

**Step No. I:**—Our stature and the influence of heredity—How to make up the heredity deficiency?

**Step No. II:**—What should the guardians do?—The foundation of one's stature is laid in childhood.

**Step No. III:**—Smoking and your stature—The nicotine in cigarettes is very injurious for health.

**Step No. IV:**—Man and the story of life—How has the neck of giraffe become long? How does the length of the various parts of the body increase or decrease?

**Step No. V:**—Our body and its structure.

**Step No. VI:**—The thyroid gland and your stature.

**Step No. VII:**—The back-bone.

**Step No. VIII:**—Dress—Its effect on the development of the body—Logic behind the selection of clothes.

**Step No. IX:**—Our diet—Substances found in our diet—What should we eat and when should we eat?

**Step No. X:**—Diet to increase your stature and to make your body strong—The diet for children—Adequate diet for adults.

**Step No. XI:**—Rest, sleep and height.

**Step No. XII:**—Massage and its effect on the increase in one's height.

**Step No. XIII:**—Sunshine, fresh air and stature.

**Step No. XIV:**—Your posture and personality Improving your posture and your point of view.

**Step No. XV:**—Which is longer?—How can the body change by the change in one's posture?

**Step No. XVI:**—How to test our posture—Examination of the various parts of the body and the devices to set the posture right—Movements to remove the defective positions—Examination of the knees—Examination of the back-bone—The defective position of the neck and the waist.

**Step No. XVII:**—Right way of sitting, walking and sleeping—Sit erect, walk erect and sleep erect.

**Step No. XVIII:**—Artificial devices of increasing one's height—From the open roof—The first and the last thing is Will Power.

---

**PART THREE: THE ATTEMPT**                    69-85

**Attempt:** The morning, the mid-day and the evening.

**Morning: Five movements for men.**

1. Running on the spot. 2. Touching a mark on the wall. 3. Boating. 4. Exercise of the waist. 5. To make the shoulders and the body flexible.

**Five movements for women.**

1. Expanding the chest—Technique 2. Jump and catch the ball. 3. Assuming the posture of a dying gladiator. 4. Exercise of the waist. 5. To make the arms and legs flexible.

**Five movements common to both men and women:** *(movement 6 to 10)*

6. Stretching the vertebral column 7. Movements while lying supported on the stomach. 8. Swinging on the rope. 9. Kick exercise—reverse. 10. The posture of rest.

**The Mid-day:** Extension movement while sitting on a chair. Straighten your waist.

**The Evening:** Sit erect, walk erect and sleep erect, think high, climb high and go ahead!

---

**PART FOUR: THE SOLUTION**                    87-95

Your questions and our answers.

*Appendix: Useful Charts*                    **96-104**

# The Programme to Increase Your Height and Improve Your Posture

## PART ONE

## THE PROBLEM

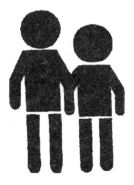

# The Problem

## Short stature–A curse

Many years ago (in the seventh decade of the 20th century) the dwarfs started a country-wide movement in Australia to provide good facilities for themselves. The short-statured people of Australia and New Zealand had participated in it by coming from every nook and corner. Their parents, too, participated in this conference to tell the people about the hardships and difficulties which their sons and daughters had to face on account of their short statures. The chairman of the conference, Whitker, who himself was a short-statured person (dwarf), told the participants that on account of being short-statured, they had to experience many difficulties in getting employment. The result was that they had become a redundant part of society.

The curse of short stature is being experienced very seriously in every corner of the world. Be it business, or high government service, only tall persons or candidates of average height are selected for the jobs. Tall stature has almost become an important condition for selection in I.P.S., Air Force or Navy. On several occasions, even in a personal sphere, short-stature stands in the way of getting a suitable partner in life of one's own choice. Several examples have come to light in France, Britain and America, where the beloved refused to marry a youngman who had a short stature. Such cases are also there when a beautiful woman had to wait for the whole of her life for marriage due to short stature.

## Short stature–An all pervading problem

(1) A youngman, Munni Lal, writes, "As I am short statured, I could not be selected for the Army."

11

(2) The son of a farmer has to say, "As I am 145 cm only in height, I could not be selected for the job."

(3) A graduate complains, "I have passed B.A. in first class. I have appeared in several tests for getting a job, in which I usually pass. But I am rejected at the time of interview as I am of a short stature."

(4) A young woman, who is called "Munni" by the members of her home, says in despair, "I am beautiful to look at. I belong to a good family, but my height is short. Hence I am experiencing difficulty in getting a suitable match.."

(5) A husband speaks thus to express his difficulties, "My wife is healthy and of a good height. I look short before her. Hence we feel shy to walk together."

(6) A teacher expresses his sorrow in the following words, "I am a teacher, but when I am in my class, I get lost amongst my students for I look short, as my stature is short. When my students see me, they smile within themselves sarcastically. This hurts me, but I cannot help it."

(7) An adolescent speaks to express his grief as follows, "I am a student of High School. But I look just half before my class fellows. All laugh at me and call me a 'dwarf'. I am unable to understand as to what should I do?"

(8) A bright girl-student says, "The stature of my mother is short and my father is tall. I have gone on my mother and my stature is short and my body is stout. I am studying in B. Com., but due to my short stature, my future appears to be dark."

(9) "When I was of a small age, I looked very thin. The height too did not appear to be short. After my marriage, I have become flabby. Now I am thirty eight years old and my stomach, too, has bulged out and the waist also appears to be bent. Now I appear to be of a very short stature. My friends call me "Chotu Ram" and laugh at me. How has this happened? I fail to understand."

(10) "My parents are of a good stature. My brothers and sisters are of a good height. But I do not know as to why

12

I am of a short stature. I am not fat, but all call me "fatty". Is there no hope for me?"

The above are some of the samples taken from the letters received by post. Each one has his or her own problem. But what is common to all these is that they have only one complaint, that their height is small or their stature is short. Had their height been a little more, they would have been much better.

## Stature and our point of veiw

Certainly we agree with many of our friends that their short stature is definitely a handicap in their progress. Had they been a little taller, they would have been more successful in their lives. But we are unable to agree with their words of sorrow and disappointment. We do not agree with their view that there is no hope for them. On the contrary we believe cent per cent that if they try with firm determination, they can certainly increase their height. On this our readers express several complaints, the gist of which is that their height is short, their personality looks poor, they lack in self-confidence and that they feel shy in the presence of others.

Our reply to all such complaints is just one. You may be a woman or a man, a child, a young man or an adult; *if you follow our programme systematically, you can certainly increase your height, that is to say that by improving your gait and posture you can also improve your height.*

## The opinion of doctors and our programme of improving the stature

If you consult doctors, they will say that the height of a man does not increase beyond a particular age. Their opinion is that height cannot increase towards the feet after a particular age. Further, when a person attains a certain age, the height cannot increase even through the backbone. But we are proud of our success and we want to repeat our statement before you that by following our progamme on "INCREASING YOUR HEIGHT AND IMPROVING YOUR POSTURE", you can observe its good results. What is self-evident needs no proof.

13

## The programme on increasing your height and improving your posture

It is not necessary to explain the meaning of our programme entitled, "Increase Your Height and Improve Your Posture". As the name itself suggests, by following this course, you can, like several other persons, remove the defects of your gait and posture and make your personality more attractive and charming.

The programme, "Increase Your Height and Improve Your Posture", is a French formula, and it has been successfully followed in Europe and America. Looking at its hopeful results, the author is convinced of its success and has full faith that the programme can be very popular and successful in the Asian countries in general and in such a big country as India in particular.

## The basis of our programme

The author has a firm faith in the principle of development. The development in the living world has taken its form on the basis of the power of determination and the continued efforts of a living being. Originally, the fish and the bird were living beings of the same class. The bird made constant efforts to fly, so it developed into a flying living being. The fish swam in water, so it developed into a 'swimming' being. The ancient man was a living being walking on four legs like an animal. He started using his front legs as hands and the result was that their structure changed slowly as compared to his hind legs. And a time came when the shape of his hands totally differed from the shape of his feet. How did this happen? It happened due to the will-power of living beings. And you are a full fledged man, the best of the living beings, (who direct and change the surroundings according to their requirements)– What can you not realize, if you so desire?

From the examples given above, it is clear that the development of bird and fish and from the ancient man to 'man' is the result of prolonged activities and has taken considerable time. You can ask as to how does it prove that the height can be increased due to a little effort on our part? The author has to point out that long-term efforts are not needed to increase one's height. The reason for this is that you want to increase your height by a few inches alone and are keen to change your gait and posture so that you may improve your personality and make it more attractive. Hence you can certainly achieve the desired benefits, by following our programme and adopting the techniques laid down therein.

## How can height be reduced or increased?

The form or shape of the different parts of our body can be modified by making efforts according to our will. There is a custom amongst the Indian Adivasi women or Bedouins to put on silver anklets or those made of bronze. On several occasions these ornaments cover more than half the leg of a woman. There is a custom amongst certain tribals to put on armlets. If we see those parts of the body where ornaments are put on, we shall find that the shapes of the parts of the body of such persons are modified according to the ornaments that they put on. The pressure is quite visible on the place where armlet is put on. The rest of the arm remains normal. What does it show?

In China the small feet of girls are considered to be signs of beauty. Hence their feet were kept in small iron frames to make them look small. Consequently, their feet remained 'small as compared to other parts of their body. All of you must be aware of this fact. On the contrary, the feet of those children who are players and who do not put on shoes and move barefooted, become large as compared to the feet of those children of the same age-group, who put on shoes.

Several centuries ago, there was a practice in Burma and Ceylon to enlarge the neck of a person by fixing an iron spring on the portion of the vertebral column just below the neck. This practice is in existence in certain places even today.

*What does all this prove? That if we make efforts, we can mould the parts of our body, increase or decrease them, in accordance with our will.* But when we are going to increase our height, we must take care to see that it remains proportionate.

15

## What is the meaning of proportionate height?

It is possible that we may increase our height too much by making use of artificial aids. For example, let us take the case of a person who increases his height by two feet. Will it be possible for him to maintain the remaining parts of his body strong in the same proportion? Our view is that the enlarged part of the body will not develop properly, the bones of these (enlarged) parts of the body will become weak and and their capacity to endure will also be reduced. We have prepared our course keeping this point in view. *We are proud to mention that our course is free from any harm to the body. The development of the body takes place side by side and it becomes strong. The most important thing is that no artificial aids have been utilized in our course. It is based on a natural technique.*

Hence we think it desirable to mention that the goal of increasing the height should, in usual circumstances, be fixed at increasing it by a few inches only. Only this much is possible by following the natural technique.

## What is the ideal height?

There has been a difference of opinion in different countries and at different times, regarding the ideal heights of men and women. The height is very much related to the climate of a country and also to the heredity of a person. This is the reason why the standards differ from one country to another. There is one standard in Greece, another in Europe and quite different from these in America. So the standard varies in Asia. The standard in India is different from that of Iran, while the standards of China and Japan are quite different from these.

In England, France and America, the average height of a man varies from five feet to six feet and four inches, while the average height of ladies varies from four feet nine inches to six feet. In Asia, the average height of an Indian is slightly below the average height of European countries, while the height in China and Japan is much less than what you find in India.

The artists, the artisans and the scientists also differ very much from each other regarding the conception of 'Ideal Height'. The scientists lay great emphasis upon the development of physique, but the artists lay greater emphasis on 'beauty' and 'symmetry'. In our opinion, both the views are correct and have their own importance. Hence both the points of view have to be kept in sight while planning to increase one's height.

The Greek standard is that the height of a man should be eight times the length of his head. The modern artists point out that the stature of a man should be seven and a half times the length of his head.

If the length of the head of a man is nine inches, his height should be five feet and ten and a half inches. This is called the ideal height of a man according to the Greek standard. In the same proportion, the height of a woman is considered to be ideal if it is five feet and five and a half inches. The form or shape of the arms, hands, neck, thighs and feet should also be in the same proportion.

## How to establish an ideal symmetry in the various parts of the body?

Such an ideal proportion of the various parts of the body is seldom visible in the ladies and gents around us. But that need not disappoint us. Here we need firstly the 'KNOWLEDGE' about the new technique and SECONDLY TO BRING INTO PRACTICE THE SPECIAL MOVEMENTS SUGGESTED ON THE BASIS OF THE NEW TECHNIQUE.

In the next two parts (1) Knowledge and (2) Attempt, we have given the basic knowledge regarding stature and have explained the ways and means to increase one's height. Any individual can increase his height by following these movements daily and regularly.

OOO

# The Programme to Increase Your Height and Improve Your Posture

## PART TWO

## THE KNOWLEDGE

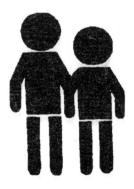

# The Knowledge

## STEP NO. I

### Our stature and the influence of heredity

Though we are not in a position to say anything definitely about 'heredity', yet we are also not in a position to deny the fact that the physical features of a man or a woman resemble those of his ancestors to a certain extent. From this it should not be taken to be obligatory that in case your parents are tall, you will also be tall, or that the offspring of short-statured parents will necessarily be short-statured. It is not essential that such a phenomenon will occur, but it is also true to say that it is often seen that the sons/daughters of a short-statured person are also short.

The scientists are busy in serious research on the basis of the results of heredity.

But this truth has created difficulties in their way of arriving at some positive conclusion, that the sons and grandsons of short-statured parents are seen to be tall, but again in the

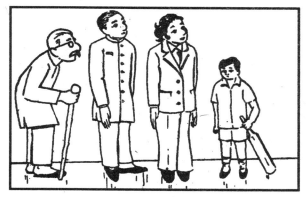

*The son, the father, the grandfather and the*
*great-grandfather—all short-statured.*

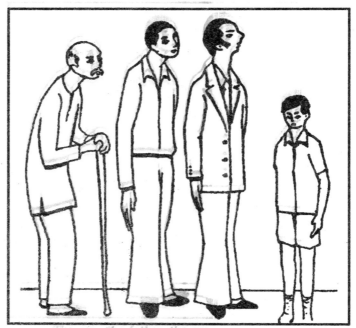

*The son, the father, the grandfather and the
great-grandfather—all tall.*

third or fourth generations, the offspring are short-statured. Heredity thus is very much shrouded in mystery. Not only height, but also complexion, posture and voice are found to resemble the complexion, posture and voice of their father, grandfather or great-grandfather.

We have observed people of various races in different countries. The Chinese, the Japanese and the Burmese are of one pattern and resemble one another. The Indians, the Pakistanis and the Iranian belong to a different pattern. The Europeans are fair-coloursed and of a different type, while the Africans are totally different from the previous ones. It is correct that their complexion and shape very much depend upon the atmosphere and environment and also the seasons or their country. But none can deny the fact that sufficient differences are visible in the castes, sub-castes, tribes and families of the same country. Differences are also visible in the inhabitants of the different states within a country. We have seen that tall and thin persons belonging to a single caste resemble their ancestors.

But from this inference you should not think that since your parents and ancestors are tall and strong, you will become tall automatically. If you are growing tall, it is all right. *But if your height is not increasing, you must pay attention to it.* If the growth of your stature is stopped, efforts should be made to reinforce the growth continuously. You should consult an expert to find out its reasons and the means to improve it. And if you are studying our 'Course', you should acquire knowledge about the same, timely.

## How to make up the hereditary deficiency?

If the height of your parents or elders is short, you should not be disappointed in the very beginning. The efforts should not be given up in despair. If you make efforts, you can undoubtedly overcome this deficiency, which you have inherited. Our course will offer necessary guidance to you in this regard.

Now it has been very much proved by scientific researches that traditional heredity is not as significant as the fact that any person, you and I, can increase our height considerably, by making right and continuous efforts in the proper direction, by taking proper diet and by performing right type of movements.

If you are tall by heredity, you should consider yourself to be lucky. *You should maintain this good luck by walking straight and maintaing a good posture by regular practice.* Thus you may make further efforts to increase your height.

But unfortunately, if you are short-statured by heredity, you should get rid of nervousness and start making efforts to become tall. Give adequate exercise to your body parts every day. *Do not bend your legs while you lie down, but lie straight while you sleep. Before you get up in the morning, you should yawn in a proper way and have an exercise of deep breathing.* In a few days you will observe that all these activities will produce a favourable effect upon you towards increasing your height.

23

# STEP NO. II

## What should the guardians do?

It is the duty of parents and guardians to see that during childhood, the development of a child is taking place correctly. If they find that the size of the body of the child is not growing properly, they should take care to see that the child does not lie in a small cradle or in a small perambulator in an uncomfortable position. On the contrary, the child should be made to lie on the bed in the open or in a big perambulator, where it can stretch its hands and legs properly. The growing child should get an opportunity of lying and playing freely on green grass under the sun and the blue sky.

Some parents make their children sleep on a single bed. All the parts of their body do not get an opportunity of developing properly, when children sleep together on one bed. Consequently they become short-statured. Hence the children should be made to sleep SEPARATELY ON DIFFERENT BEDS.

## The foundation of one's stature is laid in childhood

The child can grow properly during its childhood under the supervision of its parents. The child whose development takes place properly in the beginning, grows into a tall and well-built adult. It can, therefore, be inferred that if the good, the attentive and the educated parents take proper care, their offspring can also grow into well-built and tall adults.

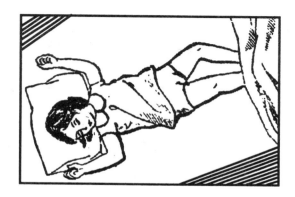

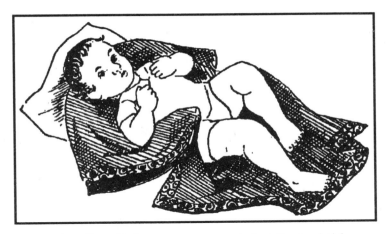

Undoubtedly, all the parents want that their children may become tall and possess an attractive personality. But only those parents can achieve their goal, who can back their desires with the right type of efforts.

## And what is this effort?

You may ask a hundred times as to what is this effort, but our reply will be one and the same. *While the child is in the growing stage, take every possible care to bring it up properly.* Put your child in the open on a mat and afford it an opportunity to move its hands and legs freely, while lying on its back.

If the ground on which the child is lying down is hard and even, it will be able to do bodily exercise by moving its hands and legs. Thus while it grows into an adult, its body will become proportionate, soft and modifiable.

On the contrary, several mothers, out of excessive affection, make their children sleep on a bed having thick cushion. Some of them think that the cushion is a sign of their affluence and assume that as their child is one in a million, why should it be made to suffer any trouble? And so they make their children sleep on a bed having thick cushions, in an uncomfortable position. You can very easily imagine the consequences.

Yes, you have correctly guessed–the child cannot develop properly. Even when the child has grown up, its body remains under-developed.

## Student period and the evil effects of wrong posture

In countries like India, when the children grow, they usually go to school. The children of average parents (who get admission in Government Schools) usually come again in an unwholesome atmosphere. They are kept together in a school. In the classrooms there is usually an insufficient light and in many cases no desks are provided to the children to work. And even in the institutions where desks are provided, they are often smaller than the size of children. Besides, there is insufficient light and air. *Such an unnatural atmosphere casts an unwholesome effect on the development of a child.* The bones are flexible during childhood. This is the age when the body grows. In such a condition, the necks of children often bend on one side and there appears to be a hunch in their backs and their waists also shrink inwards. The knees of several children start bending downwards and the sides of the backbone develop unnatural curves.

*When the wrong posture becomes a part of the nature of a child, the development of his body, when he comes of age, does not take place properly.* Those amongst you, who have become short-statured on account of bad posture should ascertain the following:

1. Did you not sleep in your childhood with your brothers and sisters on a single bed in an uncomfortable position?
2. Did you not sleep on a small bed so that you had cultivated the habit of bending your legs while sleeping?
3. Have you not developed the habit of sitting in a crouch position?
4. Did you not develop the habit of leaning forward while walking, in your student days, due to heavy load of your school bag?
5. Did you not lean forward while reading?
6. Did you not take adequate part in games in your school?
7. Have you not cultivated the habit of reading while lying in bed?

You will find that most of these defects existed in you. We would like to add here that if you are short-statured or your posture is defective, or your personality is not attractive, there is one reason for all these shortcomings, that you have *cultivated wrong habits, on account of which your stature has remained short, or if it is not short, it looks short.*

The only remedy to improve your height is that you should bring improvement within yourself even at this stage and try to give up the bad old habits, gradually. The older a habit, more is the time taken in giving it up. This does not at all matter, for even Rome was not built in a day. Make a fresh beginning and proceed towards improvement step by step.

# STEP NO. III

## Smoking and your stature

In the opinion of a physiologist of Chicago, tobacco contains nicotine, which is so poisonous that if 1/400 oz. of it is injected into the blood of a man, he will die. One third part of this quantity is always present in each cigarette. The heartbeat increases due to nicotine. The heart of a smoker has to beat 30,000 times in twenty-four hours. From this it is gathered that nicotine is a poisonous substance. *Due to constant smoking slow poison accumulates in the body. The lungs are consequently affected and digestion is also disturbed. The rickets of the chest increase and memory is also affected.*

*Warnings have been given against smoking, from time to time, in the various spheres of society. But the smokers laugh at these warnings and do not care for them.* They do not think them to be worthy of consideration. In the buses and trains we often find it written: 'SMOKING PROHIBITED'. Even in offices, cinema halls and factories and also at places of public interest, such a prohibition is notified. You should have thought over the reasons for the

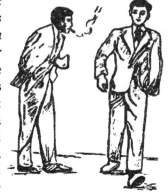

27

same. The main reason underlying this warning seems to be the need for protection from fire. There is, however, another reason, and it is this that smoking is considered to be anti-religious and anti-moral in certain places.

Besides this, those people who do not smoke find faults and faults alone in smoking, while those who smoke, dwell upon its need and point out that it creates in them a mood (to work) and helps clear their bowels.

But here we are not concerned with the other advantages or disadvantages of cigarettes. We only want to know whether cigarette smoking is at all concerned with the increase or decrease of our stature.

We are not to analyze here the cigarettes scientifically and to put up before you a long list of poisons found in them and to startle you thereby. We only want to state briefly that the cigarettes contain certain poisonous elements, which very much hinder the development of the body, particularly during adolescence. Smoking not only badly affects the lungs of a person, but there is always a fear of 'cancer' and the growth of the stature is also retarded. This is the conclusion which is derived from the latest scientific researches. *All the scientists also agree with the inference that the nicotine present in cigarettes is very much harmful for health. Hence the people who want to increase their height are advised to get rid of this habit as early as possible.*

# STEP NO. IV

## Man and the story of life

The scientists believe that the origin of life on earth began with organisms having only one cell. Man emerged after twenty billion years from the time of the origin of life. In the beginning, man was also an organism (animal) like a monkey walking on four legs. The chimpanzees and the gorilla resemble man in form and belong to the category of monkeys and make use of their fore-legs as their hands.

The scientists are of opinion that man stood up on his legs about two lakhs years ago. At this stage of development, the main burden was placed on the backbone of a man.

(Our topic is related to the stature of a person, which is mainly related to the backbone.)

The form in which our hands and feet exist today, were unlike those which existed in very ancient times. The present shape has emerged after thousands and lakhs of years of effort. Our continuous efforts in the present will determine the physical development of future generations.

## What does it prove?

*It goes to prove that we can develop in the direction in which we want to, by making efforts in that direction and also on the basis of having a strong will.*

Now let us consider this point with reference to one's stature. You can increase your height, provided you make positive efforts. There is no doubt about it.

## How has the neck of giraffe become long?

The skeletons of giraffe of ancient times go to show that their necks were short and not so long as you find them today. How have they become so long?

The scientists think that the main nourishment of giraffe was the leaves of trees and it was on this that they survived. When they had consumed the leaves of all the trees, they started eating the branches of trees existing at greater heights. For this they had to stretch their necks to a great extent. Due to constant stretching of their necks, they became long. The giraffes having long necks gave birth to offspring having long necks. Thus possessing a long neck became a hereditary characteristic of a giraffe. And now we see that the neck of a giraffe is so tall that it is not possessed by any other living being.

*The example of the giraffe goes to prove that if we make efforts, we can increase the height of our body.*

## How does the length of the various parts of the body increase or decrease?

The structure of any part of our body is closely related to its function. If the function of any organ changes, then its structure will also undergo a change. Conversely, if the structure of any part undergoes a change, its function also changes. If a man takes exercise every day, the muscles of those parts of the body, which perform the relevant movements, become strong. The more you take work from an organ, the form and shape of the muscles of that organ gets enlarged proportionately and they also become strong. On the contrary, the muscles of those organs of the body which are not used, are gradually reduced in size and even their natural form slowly disappear.

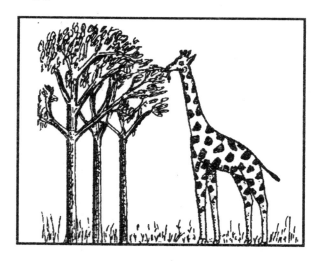

# STEP NO. V

## Our body and its structure

The structure of the human body is very complex. Our body is made of innumerable cells. These cells are divided into a number of groups which are called tissues. Certain tissues form the external surface of the body, while others join other tissues. Some tissues go to form 'muscles' while others form 'nerves'. An organ is formed by a group of tissues. These organs can be made strong and be developed by giving proper exercise and movements to them.

As you are aware, there are nine main organ systems in our body. Their brief descriptions are given below:

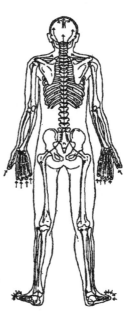

(1) The Skeletal System:— It provides the skeleton for the body. There are many bones in it, whose joints are interconnected with several connecting tissues. Thus a man can direct the various movements of his body. The backbone has a special place in the human skeleton. (it is also closely related to the stature of a man.)

(2) The Muscular System:—Its function is to help in the performance of movements of the different parts of the human body such as head, neck, arms, trunk, legs etc. It performs the function of blood circulation and sends the food in the food pipe of the body. All the activities of our body are governed by this system.

(3) The Digestive System:—Its function is to digest the food which generates energy. (The undigested food is also passed out in the form of stool through this system.)

(4) The Respiratory System:—To get energy from the food that is digested, oxygen is necessary. This system helps in the procurement of oxygen. It also helps our body to send out carbon dioxide gas from it.

(5) The Circulatory System:—This system is responsible for sending the energy procured from the nourishing elements of our food and the oxygen procured from the air, to all the parts of the body. All the cells of our body require energy and oxygen. Its circulation takes place through blood. The blood, the blood vessels and the heart–all three combine to form this system.

(6) The Excretory System:—Its main function is to send out the refuse and the useless matter out of our body. The kidneys, ureter and urinary bladder form this system. (The urine is passed out through this system.) Other parts of the body also assist in sending out the waste matter e.g. perspiration from the skin and sending out carbon dioxide gas from the lungs.

(7) The Reproductive System:—The organs which form this system are different in men and women. The reproductive organ of the male consists of the penis and the testes, while reproductive organ of the female consists of ovaries, uterus and other parts.

(8) The Nervous System:—It exercises a check over the functions of the different parts of human body. The brain, spinal chord and the nerves form this system.

(9) The Endocrine System: —'Endocrine' means secreting internally. This system mainly consists of certain glands, which secrete fluids, which get directly mixed up in the blood. These secretions are called 'hormones' and the glands secreting them are also called 'ductless glands'. The important glands are thyroid, adrenal, pituitary and the pancreas. Though there are several systems in our body, yet all of them function together. *The thyroid gland is mainly connected with the development of the body and the stature of a person.* We will discuss it in brief in' the next step.

# STEP NO. VI

## The thyroid gland and your stature

Yes, as we have already told you the thyroid gland is an endocrine gland on account of which the hormone directly mixes with the blood. It is a ductless gland.

The thyroid gland is associated with the weight of a person. On the basis of recent researches, the experts have arrived at the conclusion that the activity of the thyroid gland creates an unprecedented increase in the height of a person in young age. Nevertheless, it is true that in the phenomenon of increase in stature, other glands too have their role to play. Even then this can be definitely stated that if this gland does not function properly, the development is not normally possible.

According to experts, "It is very difficult to study the general functions of this gland in an average individual. To understand its function, the best course is to observe the defects which are found (in a human organism) when this gland does not function properly or when it is removed from the body of a person. In that condition, the growth of the bones is stopped or the bones are deformed or mis-shaped. The sexual maturity of a person becomes slow or is stopped. The skin becomes dry. The muscles grow weak and fatigue occurs. Not only this, the development of the body stops, the stature remains short and a growing body too tends to become short."

From the study of the above defects, one thing becomes very clear that the thyroid gland affects all the cells of the body and, therefore, it is very significant.

Now let us look at its reverse. If the thyroid gland becomes hyperactive, the result will be just different. The heart-beat increases, the appetite increases all at once, but after having taken food in an unusual quantity, the person becomes dull all of a sudden. The person feels great energy and enthusiasm in him, and becomes very much restless. The skin becomes moist. The temperature of the body increases, and the quantity of glucose in it becomes more than normal.

It need not be said, that the claim of increasing the height can be made in such circumstances, but the person should be treated by an expert physician, otherwise the desired results will not be forthcoming.

In the nineteenth century, there were many fields in the inland regions, which were called 'Goitre Zones', for the inhabitants of such places mostly suffered from the hypo-activity of the thyroid glands. They were administered iodine, which led to the disappearance of the disease, and their normal growth began again in its natural form.

If you are anxious to increase your height, follow our course according to the technique outlined and you will find that you have improved a lot and you are on the path of progress.

# STEP NO. VII

## The backbone

In the backbone of the human body, there are 33 vertebrae. Each vertebra has a hole in it, resembling a ring. The vertebrae are joined together and form a continuous hollow tube in which the spinal chord is lodged. The vertebral column can be divided into five parts:

(1) The Cervical Region (2) The Thoracic Region (3) The Lumbar Region (4) The Sacral Region and (5) The Coccyx Region.

The upper-most part of the vertebral column forms the part of the neck which has seven vertebrae. The first and the second vertebra of the neck are joined in such a way that we can move our head in any direction that we like–forward or backward, towards the right or the left.

The second part of the vertebral column is called the Thoracic Region. There are 12 vertebrae in it. The third part is called the Lumbar Region. The vertebrae present in this part are long and heavy. There are 5 vertebrae in it.

The fourth part is called the Sacral Region. There are 5 vertebrae in it, which are separate from each other at the time of birth. Later they get joined together and take the shape of a bone in a triangular form known as Sacrum.

34

The fifth part is called the Coccyx Region. It has 4 vertebrae, which after sometime join with each other and form a Coccyx.

The backbone has a very important position in our body. It is not only the backbone of the body, but it is also the backbone of the health of a man. The stature of the man is very much related to the vertebral column. If the backbone in functions properly, the man enjoys good health. Usually when people feel pain in the back, or in the waist, they become anxious. We have outlined certain movements for the backbone in Part Three of the Book entitled 'ATTEMPT'. If you practise these movements regularly, you will find that your height is continuously increasing and the pain in the back or waist will totally disappear.

If we do not perform movements prescribed for the backbone regularly and become careless in looking after our body, and also adopt a defective posture while sitting, the backbone will develop certain curvatures. *When these curvatures increase, the stature will become short and several other defects will follow.* These defects can be easily removed only by a regular practice of the movements prescribed.

There is a spongy cushion like structure in between two vertebrae, which protects them from getting rubbed against each other, while they are in motion. When this cushion comes out from its proper place or is dislocated, there is pain in them. In that condition, one has to go to the orthopaedic surgeon and get the dislocated cushion set in its proper place.

*In order to ensure that the vertebrae and the cushions function properly, the backbone should be massaged daily with oil. This will not only make the vertebral column healthy, but also lead to its development.*

# STEP NO. VIII

## Dress and its effect on the development of the body

Perhaps you have not cared to observe that some ladies and gents appear to be taller and more impressive, when they put on proper dress while there are other persons, whose stature is not short, but they look short statured for they do not put on proper dress. Its main reason is their selection of proper or improper dress.

These days the fashion of putting on tight dresses seems to be on the increase. People put on tight shirts, tight pants, tight waist-coats or jackets. The ladies put on tight shirts, tight 'salwars' or tight blouses. If you look at their shoes, you will find them to be tight. If you ask its reason they would say, "It is the fashion these days."

## What is fashion?

To put on clothes, as other people do, is called fashion. It is not very good for the people to remain distinct from the rest knowingly, but blind imitation is something very bad.

As far as the fashion of putting on tight clothes is concerned, it is defective. (Luckily the attention of certain people has gone in this direction and an opinion has grown against it.)

The development of the body of a human being takes place in the same way as the growth of plants and trees. While planting trees, we take care to see that their roots get sufficient space to grow. Their roots should get sufficient water from the ground to suck. They should get sufficient air and sunshine. Only then it is possible for the plant or tree to grow and yield fruits and flowers.

*If you are in the habit of putting on tight clothes, your body cannot grow properly.* It is not a fact that tight clothes are just uncomfortable. Our body is continuously growing. If we afford proper opportunity to it, it will grow. This can only happen when we put on such clothes which would afford freedom to move all the parts of our body.

*The growth of the legs of such children is retarded, who put on tight pants or tight 'churidar payjama'. In the same way, the girls should not put on tight clothes.*

It is harmful to put on tight banyians, underwears, tight shorts, tight shirts, bush-shirts, coats and waist-coats. They hinder the growth of chest, thighs and arms. Tight cuffs and collars are also harmful. The growth of the neck stops, if tight collars are put on. The growth of the wrists is also hindered on account of tight cuffs of shirts.

## Logic behind the selection of clothes

People of average stature and physique should neither put on very tight clothes nor those very loose. But fat people can be advised to put on a little tight clothes so that their corpulence may be slightly checked. From this it follows that the directions too can vary according to changing circumstances. If fat people put on loose dresses, their corpulence can further increase.

There are certain people whose legs are smaller as compared to the upper portion of their bodies. Conversely, there are people whose legs are longer and the upper portion of their bodies is smaller. In case you want to show the upper portion of your body longer than the lower, you can put on an open shirt or have your shirt outside your pant. Similarly, those people whose legs are smaller, but who want to show their lower portion taller can do so by putting their shirts inside their pants.

On contrary, there are some ladies who are unusually tall. If they do not want to show themselves very tall, they should put on loose dresses. This would make their stature look a bit shorter.

# STEP NO. IX

## Our diet

Food is absolutely essential to keep a man alive. Three types of substances are derived from the food that we take. First those which act as a fuel for our body, second those which help us to recoup the damages done to our cells and tissues. The third substance helps in the improvement of our health. The diet which gives us all the three substances is called a 'balanced diet'.

## Substances found in our diet

Our food mainly contains three elements: These are carbohydrates, protein and fat. Besides, several types of minerals and vitamins are also found in our food.

We give below a brief description of the substances found in our food:

(1) Carbohydrate–Just as an engine requires fuel to run, similarly our body needs fuel, i.e. energy, which is derived from carbohydrates.

   Carbohydrates are derived from starch and sugar in our food. Starch is derived from wheat, rice, barley, maize, pulses and potato. Sugar is derived from 'gur', glucose and sugar itself.

(2) Protein–It is found in pulses, meat, fish, eggs, milk and curd. It is very necessary for the growth of our body and increase in our height. Since the body of a child grows faster, it requires more protein than what is needed for an adult.

(3) Fats–Fats are found in oil, ghee, fish, eggs and milk. Fats give more energy to our body than the carbohydrates. We need more fats in cold weather to keep our bodies warm.

(4) Minerals–Our body needs several types of minerals. It would not be relevant here to dwell upon them in detail. It would be sufficient to mention their names. For example, calcium, phosphorus, iron, bronze, sulphur, sodium, potassium, magnesium and chlorine. Of these the first three, calcium, phosphorus and iron are essential for the development of the body, for the increase in height and for making the bones strong. Iron is necessary for the formation and growth of red blood corpuscles. These minerals are found in milk, butter, meat, eggs and green vegetables. (Those desirous of increasing their heights should take these THREE according to a fixed schedule.)

(5) Vitamins–They were discovered around 1890 by the scientists on the basis of their research. Vitamins are

found in fruits, grains and vegetables, but some of the vitamins are destroyed or reduced in quantity when the food is cooked. Hence these days vitamins are also available in the market in the form of tablets, capsules and syrup. The use and intake of vitamins is necessary to maintain the strength and the working capacity of the body. Certain diseases are also treated by the use of vitamins, where disease is the outcome of deficiency of vitamins.

Vitamins are of many kinds A, B, C, D and E. Brief details about them are given below:

Vitamin A—*This vitamin is very essential for the development of the body and the increase in one's height. It is very necessary for the strength of our bones and teeth.* The eyes also grow weak due to the deficiency of this vitamin. This vitamin also increases the resistance of human body towards disease. The children should get this vitamin in sufficient quantity, so that the development of their body may be proper and the growth of their bones and teeth may not be hampered.

Vitamin A is found in sufficient quantity in milk, butter, cheese, cod liver oil and yellow of the eggs. Carotene which is found in green vegetables, such as carrots, turnip, radish etc., creates vitamin A when it enters our body. Vitamin A is also found in sufficient quantity in the liver of animals and also in tomato.

Vitamin B—It is really a complex of 12 vitamins. It is also called B-Complex. This vitamin is found in seeds, pulses, cabbages, carrots, eggs, liver, green vegetables, milk, cheese etc. The deficiency of this vitamin gives rise to the disease called Beri Beri.

Vitamin C—This vitamin is found in greater quantity in fruits such as lemon, orange, galgal, mausami, amla and tomato. It is also found in leafy vegetables. This vitamin helps our growth to a large extent. The bones of such children, who do not get this vitamin in sufficient quantity, do not develop properly.

Vitamin D—This vitamin makes the structure of our bones and teeth strong. It is found in the oil of shark fish, liver, milk, cheese and yellow of the egg. Due to deficiency of this vitamin, one suffers from the diseases of bones and trouble in legs. Sometimes the legs of children bend due to its deficiency. Their chest shrinks and the trunk of the body bulges out. Due to the deficiency of vitamin D in young age, the bones lack in calcium and phosphorus which create a tendency in them to break.

Vitamin E—This vitamin is found in oil of the sprouting wheat, milk, meat, eggs and the whole grains. This is very essential for the maintenance of the sex-health of women.

We have a specific purpose in view in dilating upon the substances found in our diet: carbohydrates, proteins and fat. We have also told you about the minerals and the vitamins found in our food. We know that you are familiar with these details more or less, but most of you think that these are highly technical things of dietary and do not, therefore, attach due importance to them. You understand that all these things are highly complicated and are mainly related to the general health of a person and have nothing to do with the increase of the height.

Here we want to point out that you are totally mistaken. A man gets every thing from a 'balanced diet' which he needs for his proper and timely development.

## What should we eat and when should we eat?

People often enquire from doctors, as to what they should eat so that they may remain healthy. The physicians, too, are often asked this question. According to the renowned American physician, W.R.C. Laitshun, this question can be answered in two words: "Balanced Diet." He further says that there are three factors which govern our diet. First is the mental condition in which the food is taken, second is the condition of the stomach of the person and his digestion and the third, which is the least important, is the content of food which is taken. If you are excited, worried or angry, you will not be able to relish even the most nutritive and delicious food. If your

40

stomach is not empty or your bowels clean, you will not be able to digest the food that you take.

## What to eat? How much to eat?

These questions appear to be very simple but really they are complicated and have a wide range. The scientists have discovered calories in our food, on the basis of their research. They have analyzed the various calories in the different items of food and have succeeded in determining the quantity of calories found in them.

For example:—

| milk | 3/4 cup | egg big | 1 | apples | 2 |
|---|---|---|---|---|---|
| sugar | 2 teaspoon ful | onions | 4 | banana big | 1 |
| butter | 1/2 oz. | potato big | 1 | pear big | 1 |

One hundred calories of energy are provided to a person by the above items of food. An individual is advised to fix his balanced diet for the whole day accordingly. Long tables have been prepared in Western countries .on the basis of which people can determine their daily diet, according to their tastes, for the whole day. According to this scheme, the general physical worker requires 2,800 calories per day and the women staying within the house require only 2,400 calories. Those who do physical work need more calories in accordance with the physical labour that they put in e.g., 6,000 calories.

In the same way, a young man requires more calories than a fully grown up adult.

After having explained the entire position to you, we want to emphasize that it is not very easy to draw definite conclusions from the discussion of calories. Hence we should grasp the fundamental principle involved that *we should take such a diet which is a combination of all good items, depending upon the environment and the season.* The different items of our diet may be changed frequently so that all the items may be included in our diet.

41

An individual's diet schedule is proposed as follows:

**Breakfast**—Seasonal fruits, dry fruits, butter and toasts, one egg and a glass of milk.

**Lunch—**

| | |
|---|---|
| (1) Flour of wheat or rice | 250 grams |
| (2) Dal | 60 grams |
| (3) Ghee | 50 grams |
| (4) Leafy vegetables, vegetables, curd, salad and raw vegetable. | |

**Dinner**—It should be light. You should fix your menu according to your taste and economic condition.

You should take light and easily digestible food both the times. While taking your meals, your mental condition should not be surcharged with emotions or restlessness. You should take your meals in a peaceful environment and without making haste. This is the ideal way of taking meals.

# STEP NO. X

## Diet to increase your stature and to make your body strong

We have given before the scientific information about the diet of a man from which you would have learnt about the ingredients of a common diet. Now we shall give here the proper suggestions for the growth of the body, which will help you to solve your problems.

## The diet of children

Our suggestion in this regard is that the children should be given such a diet which will make their bones strong and also increase their height. To achieve this end, you should give them pulses, ghee, butter, milk and rice in sufficient quantity. If this may not be possible, you may give them some of the following items in their breakfast. These are eggs, fish, tomato, apples, grapes or almond.

At the time of lunch, you should give them the soup of boiled nourishing vegetables such as beans. On special occasions you may give them dry fruits such as dry resins and dates.

The menu of the food at night can be fixed according to their taste. The meals at night should be lighter than the one in the morning, so that it may easily be digested.

Out of the liquid diets, you may give the children barley water, ovaltine, coco, along with other fruit juices. These drinks should be taken an hour after the meals.

The parents who are desirous of developing the body of the child and increasing its height should give nourishing diet to their children. Some children do not like the pulses, rice and vegetables, but want to eat pastries, tasty and fried snacks and sweets. Some like only potato and others want to eat 'rajmah' only.

*The parents should not yield to the obstinacy of the children, in such a condition. On the contrary, they should be explained with love that when only one item of food is taken, some ingredients become excessive in body, which is harmful. When other items of food are not taken, the body becomes weak, which gives rise to a number of new diseases. We believe that the children will value your arguments and your job will become easy.*

## Adequate diet for adults

Both tall and strong and short and weak statured persons live in the same country, same state, or same village. Have you ever thought as to why is it so?

The fact is very simple. The first type of people live systematically, take proper and nourishing diet, and eat in a proper way. The people of the second type do not live systematically, and they do not take their meals in a proper way. They are ignorant of the principles of dietary. They do not even know as to what they should eat and how much they should eat.

In so far as the question of taking proper diet to increase your height and to make your body strong is concerned, you

43

should try to include in your diet protein, iodine, calcium, phosphorus and iron. Side by side, the vitamins A, B, B-complex, C and D etc., should also be taken.

**Protein:** You can have protein from pulses, meat, fish, eggs, milk and curd. Protein is also available in cashew-nut, almond-nut, groundnut, peas and beans. If more protein is needed, you may buy protein powder from the market, which can be taken with milk or water as convenient.

**Iodine:** You can have iodine from tomato, green peas, fish etc. *Iodine is responsible for the proper development of the body. It also increases the height of a person. It is also essential for making the thyroid gland strong.*

**Calcium:** If bones have not developed properly, calcium will be needed in sufficient quantity to make its deficiency good. If calcium is not, procured in sufficient quantity from one's diet, the bones themselves draw calcium from their own resources. First of all they draw calcium from the vertebral column and later from the pelvic bones. *If the calcium deficiency is not made good in time, the stature of a person remains short.* Due to calcium deficiency the vertebrae of the vertebral column become weak. Due to weight, they develop unnatural curves. As a result of this the height of a person is reduced by a few inches. Quite a number of people develop hunches of their back. *Due to calcium deficiency several defects enter the human skeleton. Hence calcium should be given to a man from the very beginning so that his height may increase as desired.*

The calcium is available in milk in its natural form, but how many people are there in our country who can afford milk for their children as well as for themselves, in sufficient quantity? So calcium tablets can be had for them from the market. Cheese and green vegetables are good sources of getting calcium.

**Phosphorus:** It is available in a good quantity in wheat, milk, meat, beans and fruits having kernel. It is an important factor in the development of the bones.

**Iron:** It is an important mineral. Good sources of iron are green vegetables, eggs, potato and meat. Grams (black)

44

when fried in an iron frying pan, yield iron in sufficient quantity.

Now we come to vitamins. In Step No. IX we have given you an introductory knowledge of vitamins. They should be taken according to one's requirement for the development of the body, strengthening of the bones and for improving the eyesight. The vitamins A, B-complex, C and D should be taken according to the need of a person. For this a good doctor or a physician should be consulted so that he may recommend vitamin tablets, which should be taken regularly.

We are indicating below in brief the conditions in which vitamins become absolutely essential:

## Vitamin A:—

(i) For developing the body and increasing one's height.

(ii) To improve one's eyesight.

## Vitamin B (Complex) :—

$B_1$—To get rid of Beri-Bery.

$B_2$—To treat the skin diseases.

$B_{12}$—To treat patients suffering from blood deficiency.

## Vitamin C :—

(i) To treat cases of scurvy.

(ii) To treat ascorbic deficiency.

## Vitamin D:—

To make the bones strong and ensure their proper growth.

## What to eat and what not to eat

It is important to know 'what to eat and what not to eat.' We should also know when to eat and how much to eat? When you will know the answers to all these questions, you will have no difficulty in maintaining an attractive posture and increasing your height.

# STEP NO. XI

## Rest, sleep and height

Most of us know the ways of working, but very few know the art of taking rest. They allow their muscles, brain and mind to function heavily during sleep. They keep on changing sides in bed and when they get up after eight or nine hours of sleep, they are not fresh for the work of the day.

Its main reason is that they do not know the technique of taking rest. It is very necessary to know the technique of taking rest, which we are describing here.

The aim of sleep is to give rest to our muscles and mind. You can give it in the following manner:

Lie down straight on a 'takhat' or on a bed made of ply wood. Have your bedding spread out evenly on it. Give rest to all the parts of your body. Take care to see that no part of

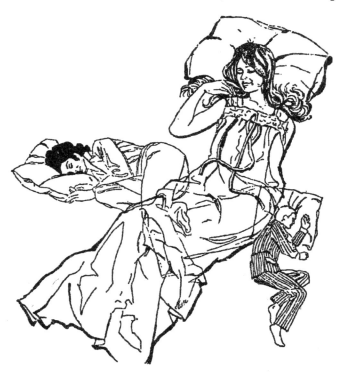

your body is made to do any extra work. Resort slowly to deep breathing. Put out the light. Close your eyes and think of the 'dark night' in terms of any dark object. Remember God and bid farewell to all the activities of the day by saying "Good Night" to them. In no time you will fall asleep.

Our body gets fatigued by working throughout the day. The cells of the body get worn out and the stature is also somewhat reduced.

*When we stretch our body to take rest, all the parts of our body get an opportunity to expand and develop. The pressure that is exerted on the backbone during the day time disappears. This affords an opportunity to the backbone to expand. Taking rest and sleeping in this way increase the height of a person continuously.*

If you are desirous of increasing your height, you should sleep for nine to ten hours a day instead of eight, while you are undergoing this course.

Always remember that 'sleep' is the main device of Complete Rest. Sufficient sound sleep acts as main tonic for increasing your height and strengthening your body. Take balanced diet and keep your digestion in order. This will enable you to have a sound sleep at night. *Sleep during the day, breathe fresh air, walk in the morning as well as in the evening and take light exercise–all these will contribute to give rest to the body and the height will go on increasing.*

It is the opinion of expert physicians of the world that we should keep our mind detached from the senses and sleep with our body fully stretched on a large-sized bed. *Allow every part of your body to get rest and see its good result.*

# STEP NO. XII

## Massage and its effect on one's height

Massage is the scientific device to make the nerves healthy, ensure proper blood circulation, and make the muscles flexible. We provide nourishment direct to the body through massage. As a result of massage, the parts of the body become active, fresh and efficient. The refuse is excreted quickly and the digestive system functions speedily. The pores of the body get opened. The stiffness caused in the muscles due to fatigue gets removed by massage. Due to its effect, the muscles become flexible, which results in their growth and development.

*Massage is really the exercise of muscles. It is directly connected with the height of a person.*

Massage has its own science. Here we will refer to it only in as much as it is related to the increase in one's height.

**(1) Massage of the back**—First of all lie down on the ground or on a hard bed supported on by your chest and stomach and let someone else massage your back. Get oil rubbed on your back. Pay more attention to the backbone.

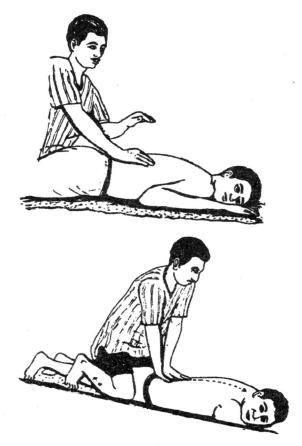

Massage should be done from upwards to downwards followed by gentle patting.

Pay special attention to both the sides of the back divided by the spine, and get both the sides massaged adequately by performing clockwise movements, stiff rubbing and patting.

*This leads to the increase in the length of the backbone which ultimately leads to the increase in the height of a person.*

(2) **Massage of the neck, arms and legs**—Join both of your hands in the shape of a bangle. The massage should begin from the upper portion of the backbone. Get the neck, arms and legs massaged by the 'twist' technique. As a result of this the unwanted elements creating fatigue will not accumulate in your muscles and the blood circulation will

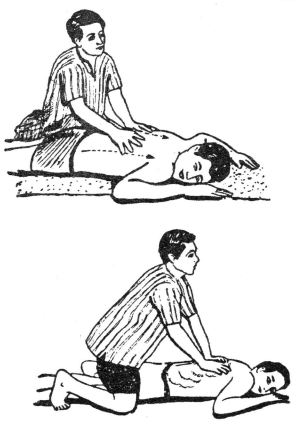

become quicker. The result is that the different parts of the body are nourished. *The massage of the neck (thyroid gland) increases the height of a person.*

Massage the legs below the ankles and the soles of your feet as well.

**(3) Massage of waist, stomach and chest**—The massage of the waist and stomach should be done by a technique involving three processes : patting, rubbing and rolling. The stomach should be kept loose at the time of massage. Let the knees lie in a standing position on the legs. The stomach should be massaged only in the morning. This massage should be done with the help of oil.

Massage can be done in a number of ways. Oil massage is the best. Besides, dry massage, powder massage, hot and cold massage can be done. People having greasy skin should resort to dry or powder massage.

The noon or evening massage can also be done with the help of powder or it can be dry.

*Thus the growth of the body takes place when it is massaged properly, rubbed effectively and patted gently.* The ladies should also massage their bodies like men and do it regularly. During pregnancy or the period of menses, the women should massage all the parts of their body except stomach and uterus.

# STEP NO. XIII

## Sunshine, fresh air and stature

Once a pair of twins was born in a hospital in Europe. At the time of birth both the children were of the same stature. The weight of one child was 3¾ kg while the other weighed 3½ kg. The first child whose weight was 3¾ kg was kept in a place where there was no sunshine. The other child was kept in the open where there was plenty of sunshine. Both were given

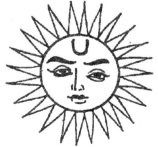

the same diet. They were medically examined after a month. It was found that the first child was of 4½ kg and the other was of 5¼ kg The child who was getting sunshine and fresh air gained 1¾ kg in weight within one month. There was another surprise. The stature of the first child became shorter, while the other child grew in stature by three inches.

This is the effect of sunshine and fresh air and reveals their importance.

*Those who live on the peaks of mountains are found to be taller in comparison to their relatives, who live in valleys.* Even in the same state it has been observed that those who work under the sun in the open fields are taller than those of their relations who live in the narrow lanes of big cities and those who work in factories. Have you ever thought as to how the offspring of the same parents are tall as well as short in stature? If one is tall, the other is short. How does the growth of one and the same person vary in different situations?

You must have understood our meaning, the reasons are sunshine and fresh air.

The famous english journalist, John Douglas says, "If some one would ask me to enumerate the three most valuable things of the world, I will say sunshine, fresh air and water." Vitamin D is present in the rays of the sun, and there is oxygen in fresh air. Water regulates the entire digestive system.

*The sunshine is the essence of all physical powers. If human body is deprived of sunshine for some time, it becomes powerless and is surrounded by a number of diseases.* Those people who work in dark rooms or underground rooms, find that their skin soon becomes pale and they suffer from anaemia and consumption.

We get light and heat from the sun. The old residents of Greece and Rome knew the importance of basking in the sun. They used to make use of the roofs of their houses to bask in the sun. Hippocrates, the father of medical sciences and Celsus were great exponents and supporters of the heat of the sun. They were of the opinion that those persons, who basked under the sun, developed great resistance against disease.

Celsus used to advise the patients suffering form nervous diseases to expose themselves to the sun.

The sun-bath should be taken in the morning sun. Put on an underwear and enjoy the rays of the sun without putting on any other clothing on the body. Slowly you will begin to perspire. The circulation of the blood will increase in the whole body. The dormant or the dead cells of the body will revive. If oil massage is also done as suggested above, you can have a complete transformation of your body in a few days. Within a few days the height of the body of a man starts increasing.

Enjoy fresh air along with the sun-bath both in the morning as well as in the evening while putting on light clothes. In the morning go to some garden and do the exercise of deep breathing. Enjoy as much oxygen as you can, inhale it and benefit your body thereby. You will find that you have become fresh.

If you feel this freshness both in the morning as well as in the evening, do you know what it suggests?

Yes, your freshness goes to prove that you are deriving the maximum advantage of the gifts of nature i.e., sunshine, air and water. If you are growing in harmony with nature, your body will naturally grow and develop.

If a plant grows when it finds sufficient sunshine and water, why will not the human being grow when it also enjoys these gifts of nature?

## STEP NO. XIV

### Your posture and personality

There is no doubt that our stature, to a very large extent, depends upon our heredity. Hence if your parents and ancestors were of a tall stature, you are also likely to be tall. But if your parents and ancestors were short-statured, the chances are that you will also become short-statured.

## Your daily routine

If the parents of some person possess a tall stature, but he himself has fallen prey to evil habits i.e. takes intoxicants, smokes or takes tobacco and possesses an irregular daily routine, neither takes his meals at the right time nor does he take adequate rest, the stature of such a person remains short.

On the contrary, there is the other person, whose parents and ancestors were short-statured, but who follows a regular daily routine himself, takes food at the scheduled time, keeps away from cigarettes, wine and other intoxicants, has fixed time for all activities such as games, walking, reading and writing, eating and drinking and resting, finds that his stature deviates from the pattern of his heredity and becomes tall and attractive.

*The conclusion that follows from this is that you should pay attention to your daily routine.*

## Your posture

The second factor after 'daily routine', which determines your stature is your posture.

Our meaning of the word posture is to find out the position in which you keep the different parts of your body while rising, sitting, walking, running or lying down. Keeping the various parts of your body in a proper position or maintaining a correct posture is as much essential for the development of your body, as it is for making your gait look beautiful and your personality attractive.

The development of the different parts of one's body takes place in the mother's womb. Sometimes, the child grows in the womb in a defective position and the structure of the various parts of the body becomes faulty. These physical deformities can be set right with the help of a doctor.

Several children do not get an opportunity of developing properly due to the mistakes committed by their mother. Several mothers are in the habit of keeping their children in their arms. When the child develops the habit of lying in its mother's arms, it starts weeping as soon as it is made to lie

53

in bed. The second mistake that the mothers commit is that when they listen the child crying, they rush to take it in their arms, though they may at that time be kneading the flour or cooking the food or cleaning the utensils. Even after taking the child in their arms, they continue with the work that they were doing. Thus the child falls into a wrong posture and its looks become defective. The result is that the different parts of the body of the child are not allowed to grow properly. On the other hand, the child forms the habit of shrinking the legs, folding the arms and bending the back which results in bending of the back as well. Such a child develops the habit of keeping the various parts of its body in a defective position. This habit is more firmly rooted in it with the advancement in age and gives rise to a defective posture, which becomes a part of its personality.

When a man or a woman crosses the adolescent period, his or her appearance and posture assume a specific pattern. His or her personality starts developing. Right posture makes a person impressive, which enables him or her to create a name for himself or herself. On the other hand, the personality of man whose posture is defective becomes gloomy and dull. Wherever he goes, he avoids company and starts losing confidence in himself. Thus your posture creates a definite effect on your personality.

## Improving your posture and your point of view

If any one forms wrong habits of sitting, rising, walking or lying, these tend to become part of his personality. The older his habit grows, firmer it becomes.

### You can improve your posture

Quite a number of persons amongst you may ask if they could rectify the wrong positions of their body; or if they could correct their posture.

Our answer would be "Undoubtedly". You can set right your posture by effort and continuous practice. The older the habit of keeping the different parts of your body in a wrong position, greater will be the effort needed to get rid of it.

So it means that our posture becomes wrong due to our carelessness or ignorace. But if we exercise a check on it and strive to practise the correct posture, the wrong posture can be set right.

Several people, on the suggestions of their friends, walk with a stiff head or a protruded chest and think that they are following the correct posture. But they are mistaken. *The posture does not become correct by making any part of our body stiff. For this we require systematic movements and regular practice. Tension is aroused in our body, when we make it or any of its part stiff artificially. But if we maintain a natural posture, our muscles become elastic and strong.* The normal posture keeps our body and its parts healthy and dynamic.

## Why is correct posture essential?

Our posture is directly related to the activities of the internal parts of our body. Wrong posture hinders the right functions of heart, lungs and circulation of blood. The curves in the spine, fallen shoulders and drooping head do not allow the heart and lungs to function properly.

You can very well realise that if the heart and the lungs do not function properly, what will be the consequences thereof. You are thinking correctly. If the blood circulation is not proper our body and its parts become weak. There is pain in certain parts of the body, while stiffness is found in others. The man becomes tired and his hands and feet become benumbed. The cumulative effect of all these will be that your posture will become all the more defective. Consequently your stature will become still shorter.

Examine your posture yourself by standing before a mirror, or let one of your friends examine it. Thereafter, start improving the position of those parts of your body which have become defective.

But here you should keep one thing in mind. Suppose you have developed the habit of walking with your head bent. To remove the wrong position of your head, you should hold it erect. But do not put all pressure on one part of your body alone. While practising the correct position.of other parts of your body, the exercise of the head should also be done. Only then you will get good results. On the contrary, if you take more work from one part of your body, or a group of muscles, you will find that you will feel much more tired and the good results which you expect will be totally absent. On the other hand, you will have to endure its bad effects.

Follow the programme of improving your posture separately, but adhere strictly to one maxim. In whatever condition you may be whether sitting, standing, walking or lying, remain erect. *Always remember that you have to sit erect, you have to stand erect, you have to walk straight and you have to lie straight.* Not only does your body become straight while you sit erect or stand erect, but your stature also looks tall, for your entire body gets an opportunity to expand.

We would like to go a step further and say that *when you try to stretch yourself fully, you go on expanding and within a short time your height begins to increase in inches and centimetres.*

# STEP NO. XV

### Which is longer?

Look at the two wires in the diagram and find out which is longer?

Probably your answer would be that the wire which is straight is longer, for it appears to be so.

But this answer is wrong, for actually the wire which is straight is of the same length which is the length of the wire that is bent. If you make the bent wire straight, you will find that the length of both the wires is the same.

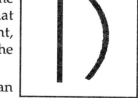

This very thing applies to the human body in relation to its different parts.

## How can the body change by the change in one's posture?

Look at the diagram in the margin. Which of the two is taller, the man on the right or the man on the left?

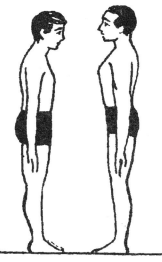

You have correctly recognised, the man on the right appears to be taller. But the two photographs are of one and the same person. Yes! You can call them two, for one photograph shows the man when he used to walk in a defective style. See how much short he used to appear at that time! The other photograph is of a later stage, when he had corrected his posture. Previously his height was five feet and six inches and now his height has increased to five feet and eight and a half inches.

Now you should understand that the stature which appeared five feet and six inches was actually taller than that. Just as if you straighten a bent wire, it appears longer, in the same way, reducing the degrees of curves in the backbone, makes it taller and straight. By constantly keeping the backbone straight, its growth has also increased.

You have not paid attention to one thing. Look at both the postures in the photograph and tell me if you find any difference between the two.

You are thinking correctly. The one man appears to be loose, easy going and middle-aged, while the other man appears to be smart and young.

But all of you know that the photograph on the left shows the former condition of the man, while the other photograph depicts the man's condition after he had improved his posture.

The man in the other photograph appears to be young, try to think out its reason. It is just this: He maintained the right posture and was, therefore, transformed.

57

# STEP NO. XVI

## How to test our posture?

Have you seen masons extending a thin rope from upwards to downwards, while constructing a house to verify the straightness of the wall constructed by them? In the same way, we can examine and verify the correctness or otherwise of our posture with the help of a thin rope, or a string.

## Examination with the help of a string

Let a string be placed from top downwards. Stand erect and let the string pass through the ear and touch the portion of your leg a little above the round bone of your ankle.

If the string passes through the middle of your ear and a little ahead of shoulders, touching the buttocks and the knee joints, and remains a little above the bone of your ankle, you should think that the position of the different parts of your body is A-One. The posture depicted in the diagram 'A' on page 59 represents the ideal condition.

Now look at diagram B and point out the defects visible therein: (1) The head is bulging out. (2) The upper portion of the back has become round. (3) There is a pit in the back portion of the waist due to its flexibility. (4) The buttocks are coming out in the back. (5) The stomach is bulging out. (6) The knees are bending forward and the feet are becoming flat due to internal pressure. This is a defective posture.

## Examination by standing close to the wall

Stand erect by the wall. Take care to see that your head, shoulders, major portion of your back, buttocks, calves of the legs, heels of the feet and arms—all touch the wall. If all the parts of your body touch the wall, your posture will be in an ideal (A-One) condition.

Your posture will be defective to the extent parts of your body don't touch the wall.

You can judge the position of your posture with the help of the following diagrams and find as to how far it is correct.

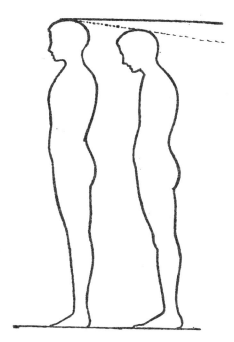

To which of these figures A, B, C or D does your posture resemble? Your posture will be of the same standard as the figure to which it resembles.

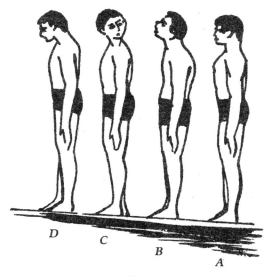

D    C    B    A

You can remove the defect existing in any part of your body by constant practice of the right type of movements.

## Examination of the various parts of the body and the devices to set the posture right

### Examination of the feet:

The right or wrong position of the feet can easily be judged by taking its print. Wash your feet and make a print on a paper or on the floor. Compare your prints with those shown on the next page. If the prints of your feet resemble the figure of flat feet, you should think that the position of your feet is defective. If your prints differ from these, you should think that your feet are healthy.

## Movements to remove the defective positions

Walk erect in the garden barefooted. Be careful to see that while walking the bridge of your feet does not touch the ground. Only the front and the hind parts of your soles should touch the ground. Walk exerting pressure on your toes. This exercise should be done both in the morning as well as in the evening. You can also walk on a clean footpath.

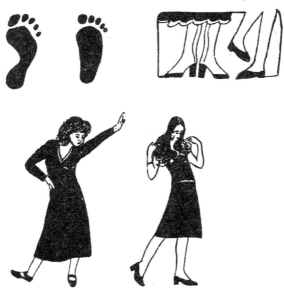

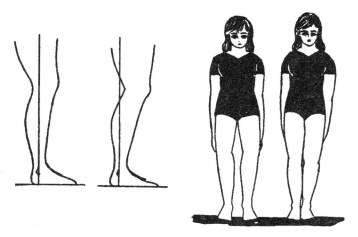

*The moment the position of your feet becomes right,*
*your posture starts improving forthwith.*

If your toes are not mobile, you can practise their movement by sitting on a chair or on a bed and picking up articles lying on the ground such as pencil, slate-pencil, chalk, small coins etc.

Your shoes play a very important role in determining the position of your feet. The shoes should neither be too tight, nor too loose. The shoes should be such as would provide comfort to the feet. The toes of your shoes should be at least one-fourth inch larger than the toes of your feet. The toes of your 'chappals' can be kept a little smaller than the toes of your shoes. Thus the toes of the feet will remain in their natural condition and well-protected.

Some people put on shoes with pointed toes, which press their toes so much that they get tired even after walking a short distance. Such shoes should be avoided.

Some ladies and gentlemen put on high-heeled shoes, without carefully thinking over it. Those persons, who are not short-statured should avoid such shoes. Those people who use them to increase their height, should not use them at all times. For putting on very high heeled shoes causes pain in the waist and makes it flexible.

61

# Examination of the knees

(1) The knees of some persons often rub against each other. (2) The legs of some children are bent in the shape of an arrow. (3) The knees of some persons are bent. These three states are the outcome of putting up with wrong positions of the different body parts for years together. They can, however, be overcome with diligent efforts.

The first and the second defect can be removed by walking regularly for five minutes, both in the morning as well as in the evening, after adopting the correct position of knees. The third type of defect can be detected with the help of a vertical line. If the line touches your ankles and passes touching the middle part of your knees, you should conclude that the position of your knees is perfectly all right. But if the knees are observed coming out of the line, you should infer that your knees are bent and defective.

# The technique of correcting the bent knees

(1) Sit erect on a chair and stretch your legs. Keep them on a stool, placed at a short distance from you.

(2) Stretch your right leg straight and remain in this position for 4 seconds.

(3) Now stretch your left leg in this very manner.

(4) Repeat this movement eight times for each leg.

*When the wrong position of the knees is corrected, the posture improves and the height increases.*

# Examination of the backbone

The backbone is really the spine of the body. The stature of the human body and its posture is very intimately connected with it. The field of the backbone can be divided into three parts: (1) the neck (2) the back and (3) the waist. The process of improving their posture is given briefly in the following slines.

**The defective position of the neck**—The neck of certain persons remain in a bent condition. To remove this defect, you should lie down on a wooden bed or a sofa (without arms) in such a way that your neck can swing easily. Bend your neck

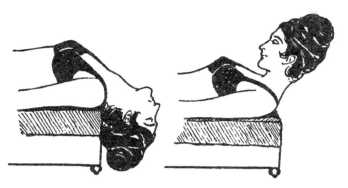

downwards as much as you can easily do. Be careful to see that this exercise is done in an easy manner and not by forcibly stiffening the muscles of the neck. If you will apply force, the desired gain will not be forthcoming, and you may be put to a loss. Now bend your neck towards your chest and try to touch your chest with your chin. Repeat this movement four times and slowly. This exercise removes the defects of posture in the neck. It tends to lengthen the neck and make it strong.

**The defective position of the back**—The back of those people, who sit for the whole day in their office or shop often tends to become double. Their backs often appear to be somewhat round. They always have some pain in their backbone. To remove this defect, they should try every now and then, to straighten their backbone while sitting, walking or sleeping.

This may take a little more time, but you can get rid of this wrong posture, by making efforts in the right direction.

To bring an early improvement in the position of the back, you should practise movement No. 5 meant for women (see part three entitled 'Attempt') one or two times in the morning, noon and in the evening as well.

*The moment the sphere of the back is set right, the height of a man begins to increase.*

**The defective position of the waist**—Those ladies, who remain busy in performing household duties or working in the office throughout the day, often complain of pain in their

63

waist. The pain in the waist is mostly due to certain inward curves of the vertebral column in the sphere of the waist. This defective position usually gives rise to certain serious shortcomings mentioned below:

(1) The head begins to bulge out. (2) The back becomes round. (3) The stomach also bulges out. (4) The knees begin to bend. In a way the whole body becomes slanting. To remove this defect in the waist, you should practise movement No. 7 (1) and (2) meant for both men and women and described in part three entitled Attempt.

# STEP NO. XVII

## Right way of sitting, walking and sleeping

Sitting, walking and sleeping are different activities of human life. While sitting and walking fall under one group, sleeping comes under a different group. Our energy is spent in sitting and walking, while we regain the lost energy in sleep.

But you will be surprised to learn that many people make their bodies work even during sleep and do not regain the lost energy and alertness. Such people do not know the correct method of sitting and walking and spend a lot of excess energy in performing these activities. Consequently they feel tired every time. Hence they should learn the correct method of sitting, walking and sleeping.

## The right way of sitting

(1) That is the proper way of sitting in which no part of the body is burdened unnecessarily.

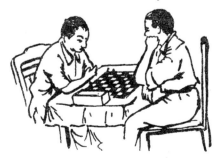

64

(2) While sitting, our back should get the right support.

(3) The height of the chair or stool should be such that undue pressure is not exerted on our thighs.

(4) There should be small chairs for children separately.

(5) The whole back should get support on the chair, right from the waist up to the shoulders. When you bend forward, the upper part of the body should come forward together as a whole and not only your neck or waist.

(6) When you feel tired, you may get up from the chair for a while. Do not become lazy and bend your shoulders or stomach in a wrong fashion, which would result in a wrong posture of your body.

There are two diagrams above, one represents a defective posture and the other a correct one. You should accordingly adopt the correct posture.

## The right way of walking

(1) The head should stand erect while you walk.

(2) The whole spine from neck to waist should remain erect, but undue strain should not be caused to any part thereof.

(3) The chest should be duly stretched while walking.

(4) The hands should not be kept inside the pockets, but the fists of the hands should be closed so that the arms can be moved freely.

(5) It should also be kept in mind that while you walk, the different parts of your body should not lie in a loose and lethargic condition. Walk systematically. It should appear from your gait as if some victorious person is coming and dominating the nearby environment.

## The right way of sleeping

While asleep our body tries to regain the energy lost during the day. Side by side the height of the body also increases during sleep. Hence we should bear in mind the following:

(1) The bed should be made of plywood.

(2) The bedding should be evenly spread on it.

(3) The pillow should be neither too thick nor too thin. This would enable the head to be raised a little above the rest of the body.

(4) The length and breadth of the bed should be of such a dimension so that we can lie straight on it and turn on both the sides, right as well as the left, easily.

(5) Two persons should never sleep together on one bed. The children, too, should not be made to sleep with others on the same bed. This creates a bad effect on the development of the height of the body.

(6) There should certainly be a window in your bedroom. This would enable fresh air to come in and you can breathe it freely.

These are very simple things no doubt, but they are of great importance. By acting on these advice, we can remove the hurdles in the way of increasing our height, while performing the various activities in our life such as sitting, walking, sleeping or waking.

*Remember the slogan: Sit erect, walk erect and sleep erect.*

# STEP NO. XVIII

## Artificial devices of increasing one's height

On several occasions due to carelessness or wrong dress, we appear shorter in height than what we actually are. On the other hand, those persons who are familiar with the art of using artificial devices look taller, when they make use of them.

'To be tall' and 'to look tall' are two different things. The first is based on truth, while the other is based on artificiality. As far as our programme of 'Increasing Your Height' is concerned, our emphasis has always been placed on the actual increase of one's height. But we cannot deny the value of these artificial devices, as they produce a significant effect on our personality. The use of these devices makes us look tall. But we must strike a note of caution in this regard: You can no doubt look taller by making use of these artificial devices and there is no harm in it, but do not use these devices to such an extent that would make you look ugly.

As the use of artificial means does not form part of our course on Increase Your Height, we are just indicating the effects of the use of artificial means on our height. If you bear these in mind, you will be able to derive some advantage from them.

(1) Put on clothes having thick and long stripes. You will look taller.

(2) Put on clothes having dark colours. This generates a feeling of a tall stature.

(3) It matters little whether you are a lady or a gentleman, you can put on high-heeled sandals or shoes and look taller. This would enable you to look taller by an inch and a half to two inches. (As we have stated earlier, high heeled shoes disturb the correct position of muscles in our waist and are at times troublesome. Hence you should put on high heels only when you have to go out.)

(4) Irrespective of the fact that you are a woman or a man, you can comb your hair in such a fashion that you can increase your height by an inch. If you are a man and you do not want to grow long hair, you can put on a hat or a cap and look taller by an inch or an inch and a half.

No doubt, to become tall is definitely more desirable than to look tall, nevertheless, these artificial devices create a wholesome effect on human personality, be it that of a lady or that of a gentleman.

## From the open roof of the first and the last thing is will-power

You have climbed eighteen steps of the edifice of KNOWLEDGE and have now reached the open roof of the building. From here you can visualize everything related to `Increase Your Height' very clearly.

You have seen that there are several factors responsible for the development of your height.

(1) You can correct the wrong position of the different parts of your body and thus improve your posture.

(2) You can give up smoking and thus cross this hurdle in the way of developing your height.

(3) You can activate the different parts of your body and thus develop them properly.

(4) You can know from human physiology the facts about the origin and growth of your body and by moulding yourself suitably, you can prepare a background for increasing your height.

(5) You can bring about radical change in yourself by putting on proper dress, taking balanced diet, adequate rest and sleep. Besides, adequate massage, sunshine and fresh air can add to your healthy growth.

(6) You can continuously increase your height by adopting the right posture in sitting, walking and sleeping.

(7) The deficiency, if any still left, can be removed by utilizing other artificial devices.

Thus you can become a successful and lucky man.

To attain this goal, the first and the last condition is: Will power. With its help you have understood your problem and have acquired 'KNOWLEDGE' about its different aspects.

And now you are going to utilize all the means to attain your goal. You are going to make the ATTEMPT to increase your height.

OOO

# The Programme to Increase Your Height and Improve Your Posture

## PART THREE

## THE ATTEMPT

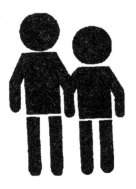

# The Attempt

You have attained sufficient knowledge regarding our programme entitled, "Increase Your Height and Improve Your Posture", which is meant for both men and women.

Now we are going to start 10 movements which you have to practise regularly every day in the morning. There should be no exception.

## The morning

Out of the ten movements, the first nine movements will take one minute each and the last movement will take three minutes. Normally a minute's rest is advised after every movement.

Take five minutes rest after performing the first five movements. Thus you have to finish this programme in a total period of 25 minutes.

Do this exercise on all the seven days of the week. The ladies should give a gap of three days during the period of their menstruation. (or till such time the blood discharge continues.) The exercise should be started again after the period of menses is over. Of course, they can perform such exercises even during the period of menses, which will not cause harm to their sexglands. They can perform the movements Nos. 4, 6, and 10 according to their own interest.

## The mid-day

The men and women, who perform desk work during the day and housewives who do sewing work in the day, should practise the movements related to making their bodies tall and straight.

## The evening

In the evening one should go to the garden and do the exercise connected with catching the ball and hanging on the rod. One or two movements related to increasing the height in a play-way fashion should be done every day.

*If these movements are practised continuously for three months, the height can increase by several inches.*

## How to perform this programme of movements?

You can derive Extraordinary benefit from this programme only when you do not give any exception. Hence perform these exercises regularly and do not give any gap. Note down briefly the movements performed by you in your diary.

But if, per chance, an exception occurs you should not lose courage. Note down the date when a gap occurs, in your diary and continue your practice thereafter. Do this week by week and month by month.

Now about the time:

The course for the morning is scheduled for 25 minutes, that of the mid-day for 5 minutes and the programme for the evening is meant for 15 minutes. Thus you have to spend only forty-five minutes in twenty-four hours to derive the desired results from our programme entitled "Increase Your Height and Improve Your Posture."

The ten movements to be performed in the morning have been divided into 25 minutes. Keep a stop-watch with you and divide your time accordingly. Allot one minute to each movement. In the beginning you can take the help of some other person to give you the relevant cautions, such as, 'STOP' and 'START'. Later on, you will yourself get the idea of time and you will be able to perform these movements freely and efficiently.

So, our good wishes are with you. Start from today the programme of Daily Exercises*.

---

*The main programme is for the morning and for 25 minutes. The mid-day and the evening programmes are supplementary.

71

# Morning

## Five movements for men
(Serials 1 to 5)

## Movement No. 1
### Running on the spot:

This movement creates warmth in the body. It is proper to begin the progamme of exercises with this movement.

Consequently, the blood-circulation increases in the whole body and all the parts of the body become alert. This movement acts as an introduction to the movements that follow. Whether you are young or old, you can perform this movement without the least difficulty.

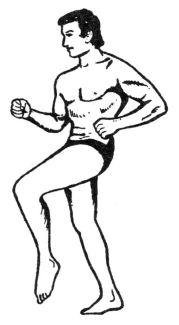

Note: Those patients who suffer from heart-trouble should not perform this movement.

### Technique

Close your fists and move one leg after another, by turns. Increase your speed slowly. Keep your hands and feet moving as much as possible, but in a natural form. Perform as many movements as you can easily do. Time: One minute.

## Movement No. 2*
### Touching a mark on the wall:

Stand erect close to the wall by joining both the legs and calves. Raise your right hand and touch the wall. Get a mark made on the wall by some one, within the reach of your hand.

---

*The first stage of this movement increases one's height.

72

Then get him make four or six marks on the wall with dark ink, each at a distance of half an inch from the previous one. Get these marks numbered.

Now stand in the same fashion as indicated before and try to touch as many marks on the wall as you possibly can. See how many marks you can touch. Repeat this exercise every day. You will find that your height is increasing.

Repeat this exercise daily, twice with both the hands, i.e., once in 15 seconds.

**Time:** One minute.

## Movement No.3*
## Boating:

(i) Stretch your legs together on the ground. Both the ankles should be kept together. Sit erect making and angle of 90°.

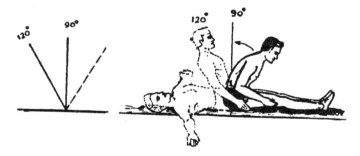

(ii) Now take the upper portion of your body towards the back and make an angle of 120 degrees. Stay for a while in this position.

---

*The first stage of this movement gives exercise to the entire upper part of the body, backbone, chest and arms.

(iii) Gradually take your body (upper portion) backwards and lie down on the ground. Stretch both of your hands towards the right and the left part of your body.

Let the muscles be left loose now and practise deep breathing.

Repeat this four times.

**Time:** One minute, 15 seconds for each turn.

## Movement No. 4
## *Exercise of the waist:

Lie down supported on the back of your body.

(i) Close up the fingers of both the hands together in the shape of a paw. Gradually bend the right leg at the knee and holding the knee with the paw bend it towards your chest. Take care to see that the lower part of the waist remains firmly on the ground and the left leg also lies straight.

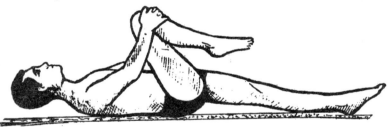

(ii) Now repeat this exercise with the left leg. In that case the right leg will lie straight on the ground.

(iii) Now practise this exercise with both the knees. You should see that the lower part of the waist remains firmly on the ground. Practise the three exercises for ten seconds each. Repeat the whole exercises twice.

**Time:** One minute.

---

*The two movements of the waist are learnt by practice. But if once the practice is acquired, it is but certain that the height of man will definitely increase to some extent.

## Movement No. 5
## To make the shoulders and the body flexible:

(i) Stand erect and keep both the legs at a distance of one foot from each other. The chest should bulge out, neck should remain erect and both the arms should be kept downwards like a perpendicular.

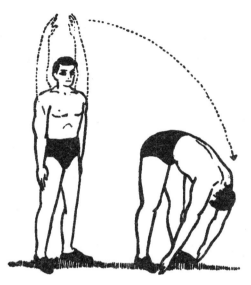

(ii) Now raise your arms upwards.

(iii) Next, bend downwards and touch your feet with your hands.

Repeat this movement four times within a minute, i.e., one movement should be performed within 15 seconds.

**Note:** Heart-patients should not perform this exercise.

**Time:** One minute.

## Five movements for women
## Movement No. 1
## Expanding the chest:

This movement expands the chest, the shoulders become strong, the posture improves, physical tension disappears and there is proper circulation of blood in the head and the brain.

## Technique

(1) Stand erect in an easy and comfortable position. Raise your arms and keep the palms of both of your hands close to your chest facing each other.

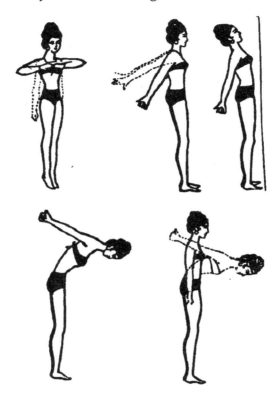

(2) Take your hand as much behind your back as possible. Close your fists and expand your chest.

(3) Take your close fisted hands as much upward towards your back as you possibly can and bend your backbone upto your waist. Keep your head forward as much as you can easily do, but take care to see that the hands remain in the back.

(4) Open the fists gradually and stand erect. Repeat it for one minute.

## Movement No. 2
### *Jump and catch the ball:

Take a ball and throw it over your head. Jump a little bit and try to catch the ball yourself. Try to catch the ball by throwing it in different directions so that the upper portion of the legs, arms and back move freely.

You can do this exercise even in the evening.

**Time:** One minute.

## Movement No. 3
### **Assuming the posture of a Dying Gladiator:

(i) Sit stretching your legs on the ground and keep your face in the front. Let the left leg be pressed below and keep the right hand on the left.

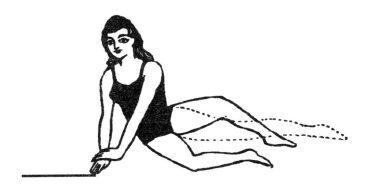

(ii) Stretch the right leg in a straight position, as shown in the diagram by the dotted line.

---

*The second movement makes all parts of the body alert and the arms too become strong.

**It is an exercise for the muscles and particularly for the legs. It accelerates the function of the creative elements of the body. This helps the growth of the stature of a person.

Now, do the exercise with the left leg and change the position of your body accordingly.

**Time:** One minute.

## Movement No. 4
## *Exercise of the waist:

Stand by the wall. Take care to see that all the parts of your body touch the wall: heels, hips, back and head. Take a deep breath and try to shrink your hips. Try to touch the wall with the hind portion of the waist. This part of the waist will touch the wall only when you will breathe deeply inside. Remember that while you breathe deeply, the stomach should shrink inside. Now, take rest by standing 'at ease'. Complete the exercise within one minute.

## Movement No. 5
## **To make the arms and legs flexible :

(i) Stand erect. Give some rest to your right hand and right leg.

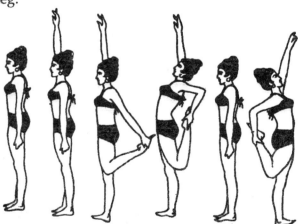

---

*The two movements of the waist are learnt by practice. But if once the practice is acquired, it is but certain that the height of a person will definitely increase to some extent.

---

**This movement makes the arms, legs and thighs flexible.

(ii) Gradually lift your right arm straight upwards. See that your head remains erect.

(iii) Bend your left leg gradually backwards and hold your left leg with your left hand. Keep your right arm upwards as before.

(iv) Bend your right hand and head a little behind and pull up your left leg a little over your back.

(v) Take rest for a while as indicated in (i) above. Repeat this exercise with the right leg, by turning in the opposite direction. (check 'right')

**Time:** One minute.

## Five movements common to both men and women
### (Movements 6 to 10)

## Movement No. 6
## *Stretching the Vertebral Column

(1) Lie down straight on your back. Leave the body loose and breathe.

Now take deep breath. Hold your breath for a while and raise your shoulders upwards. Turn your legs in such a way that both the knee-caps face each other and toe of one foot touches the toe of the other.

Release the breath slowly and bring your arms at their own place. Keep the knee-caps in their natural position. Complete this exercise within 15 seconds.

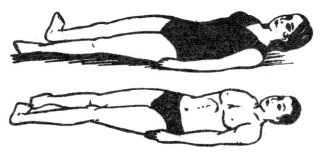

*This movement gives a very good exercise to the backbone and results in the development of the body. It is particularly helpful in increasing one's height.

79

(2) Now, lie straight on your back as you did in the first position. Breathe and let your body lie loose. Hold your breath for a while, as you did in the previous exercise, and raise your shoulders towards your head. Bend your legs in a direction opposite to the previous one. Turn your legs in such a way that the joints of the ankle touch the ground. This exercise should also be done by holding your breath. The breath should be released only after you have reached the final stage of exercise.

Perform both of these exercises twice by turn and not more. After performing this exercise, leave the body loose in a state of rest for some time.

**Time:** One minute.

## Movement No. 7
## * Movements while lying supported on the stomach:

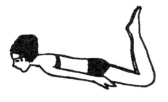

(1) Lie down on the ground taking the support of the stomach. Let your arms rest fully on the ground on both the sides of your body. Your chin should also touch the ground. Bend your legs at the knees and try to stretch the soles of your feet towards your back.

(2) Now hold both of your feet with both of your hands. Exerting pressure on them, try to raise your chin as much above the ground as you can. Leaving the legs apart, and

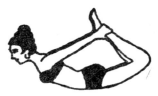

remain lying on the ground with the support of the stomach, for a few moments. In this condition only the stomach touches the ground and the chest and the thighs are raised above the ground.

Now revert to the first position. Let the arms lie straight on both sides of your body. The whole body from chin to the

---

*This movement mobilises the backbone, arms, legs, knees, stomach and chest. The blood circulation increases and the body becomes alert. Thus the posture improves, which increases one's height as well.

knees will lie on the ground supported on the stomach. The legs will be bent upwards from the knees.

Gradually straighten your legs. Breathe deeply and change the sides.

Repeat this exercise by turns. Each turn will take 16 seconds. Do it twice.

**Time:** One minute.

## Movement No. 8
## Swinging on the rope:

Fasten a rope in the iron bangle (kund) in the ceiling. Tie a small wooden rod at the other end of the rope, so that you can swing by holding it in both of your hands. Now, hold it and swing. As far as possible, keep your mouth closed while swinging. Stop in between and take rest. Swing again.Stop swinging when you feel tired.

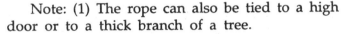

Note: (1) The rope can also be tied to a high door or to a thick branch of a tree.

(2) Weak ladies and gents can sit in a swing and perform these movements easily.

**Time:** The same one minute.

\* **Swinging on the rod**

You can swing on the iron rod fixed to a stand on the ground. The rod should certainly be at least at a height of one foot more from the reach of both of your hands.

While swinging on the rod, move your feet high with a force and give a push. This will bring speed in your swinging. If your breathing becomes fast and you start perspiring, stop for a while and take rest. Swing again after the moments of rest are over.

---

\*In both the conditions, the height increases by the arms, legs and backbone.

Even ladies can swing in this way, if they are in a normal condition. Fat persons and those suffering from heart disease should not perform this movement.

**Time:** One minute.

## Movement No. 9
## *Kick exercise–Reverse:

Stand behind a chair. Hold the upper part of the chair with both of your hands and bend forward. Raise the right leg slowly towards the back, as much as you can. Take care to see that the entire leg is lifted in the position of a straight line, without bending at the knee. Remain in this position for 5 seconds. Breathe comfortably. While performing this exercise keep your chin upwards.

Repeat this exercise with the left leg.

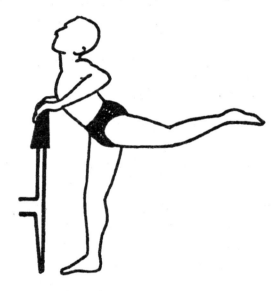

The movements of both the legs should be performed four times, by turns.

**Time:** One minute.

---

*This movement makes the backbone strong and legs get an exercise.

## Movement No. 10
## The posture of rest (*Time: One minute*):

Concentrate your attention on giving rest to each muscle of the different parts of your body. Lie down on the ground taking support of your back and leave your hands and feet loose. Keep a distance of nine inches between the ankles of both the feet.

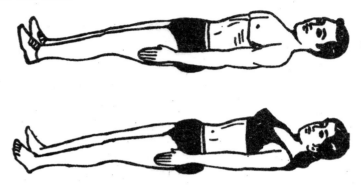

Let both the arms lie straight on the right and left side of your body comfortably and free from all tension. The hands and fingers should also remain loose. Let the head move freely on its pivot in the vertebral column. Allow your face to move in any direction it chooses. Open your mouth a little bit and let your jaw lie in any position in which it feels convenient. Keep your eyes closed and let your body lie free from all motions.

Hold your breath for a while. After some time release your breath and then breathe inwards. Concentrate your mind on rest so that the nerves may also get complete rest.

This posture removes all kinds of physical and mental fatigue. *When the body wilt get rest, its proper development will take place and the height will increase.* The fatigue caused by the performance of the earlier movements will totally disappear when you will practise this posture of rest. Hence this posture has been kept in the end of our programme after due consideration.

The practice of this posture is a bit difficult, for we have to control both our mind as well as our body in it. A man or a woman who can take up real rest voluntarily, will find his/her body always developing (and his/her height will increase as much as possible.) The reason for this is that such a person knows the secret of regaining the energy that has been spent in performing the activities of the day.

## The mid-day

Those men and women, who perform their work by sitting on the chair all the day long and those housewives, who do tailoring or sewing work at home, should perform these movements to make their body long and straighten their waist.

### Extension movement while sitting on a chair:

Make your legs straight. Also straighten your backbone from waist to neck. Raise your hands straight upwards. Do this for 30 seconds.

### Repeat it four times

This will result in the extension of the backbone. The muscles which shrink on account of sitting at one place, get an opportunity of expanding due to this movement:

### Straighten your waist:

(1) Take your left hand to your back through your waist and the right hand, over your shoulder to your back and hold the fingers of one hand with the other. Let the palms of both the hands be entangled with each other.

(2) Pull the palm of the hand below with the palm of the hand above. Thereafter pull the palm of the hand above with the palm of the hand below. Then leave the hands apart.

(3) Now, take your left hand over your shoulder towards your back and the right hand through the waist to the back and let both the hands meet each other. Now practise the movements 1 and 2 in the reverse order.

84

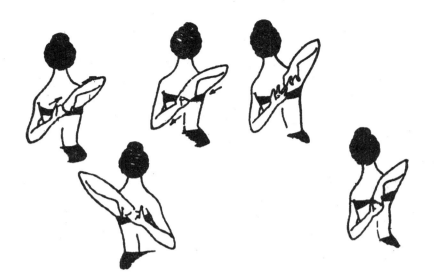

## The evening

(1) Come out of your homes for a walk in the evening.

(2) Practise the Movement No. 2 meant for women: "Jump and catch the ball." Reduce it in the form of a game.

(3) Lie down on the grass for some time, both on the right as well as on the left sides of your body. The longer you can lie on the grass, the better it would be for improving your height. When your body becomes free from tension, you should practise swinging on a rod.

Repeat the following motto while practising this exercise:

**Sit erect, walk erect and sleep erect,**
**Think high, climb high and Go Ahead!**

# The Programme to Increase Your Height and Improve Your Posture

## PART FOUR

## THE SOLUTION

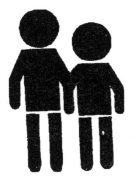

# The Solution

*(Your Questions and Our Answers)*

**Question:**    "The height of a man increases only till the age of 21 years." What is your view about this opinion of doctors?

**Answer:**    Yes, according to human physiology the bones of a man get closely joined together near about the age of 21 years. Hence they do not develop further. But it is not absolutely correct to say that the height of no one increases beyond the age of 21 years. It is correct to say that when one reaches this age, the development will be visible only above or below the back and not in the legs.

**Question:**    Should we infer thereby that the length of the legs does not increase at all beyond the age of 21 years?

**Answer:**    No, there are several persons whose height has increased even after this age.

**Question:**    I am forty years old. Can my height increase even now? If so, how?

**Answer:**    Undoubtedly, your height can increase even at this age. On several occasions your body shrinks on account of wrong postures and defective positions of the various parts of the body, and you start looking short. You can improve your height by improving your posture. Besides, your height can increase by taking good and nourishing diet which can make you strong and sturdy. Adequate rest, sleep, massage and sun-bath also contribute towards the development of your body resulting in the increase of your height. By acting upon the suggestions given in this book and following the programme entitled "Increase Your Height and Improve Your Posture", you can observe its outstanding effect on your body.

**Question:** When I measure my height, I find it to be four feet and nine inches. But it does not appear to be that much. What is its reason?

**Answer:** You do not maintain the right posture of your body. Follow the instructions given in Part II of this book dealing with "KNOWLEDGE" in the chapters relating to the maintenance of the correct posture of the different parts of your body. By doing so, your gain will be unprecedented.

**Question:** How does my height come out to be full when measured?

**Answer:** When you stand erect, your height comes out to be full. But while sitting or walking, you lean forward, so you appear to be short. Hence you do not look the height that you actually are.

**Question:** What is the proof that the backbone is flexible?

**Answer:** As it is self-evident, it does not stand in need of any proof. The backbone extends from the neck to the lower part of the waist. As the backbone is flexible, you can bend your neck, back and the waist according to your will. Let us give you a proof. If you measure a man in a standing position form neck to waist, the length will be 26 inches. But if you ask the same man to bend forward towards his feet and then measure the length of his back, you will find it to be 28 inches. This is due to its flexibility.

**Question:** The head of my father is bulging forward. Why is it so? Tell me how to remedy it.

| | |
|---|---|
| **Answer:** | Is it not so that the eyesight of your father is poor, on account of which he has cultivated the habit of protruding his neck forward, while reading? Whatever may be the reason thereof, in case he wants to set it right, he can do so by constant practice of the movements suggested in Step No. XVI of Part II. |
| **Question:** | I am taller than my younger sister by two inches. But every one says that I appear to be shorter than her. How can it be so? |
| **Answer:** | A curved wire can be more in length than a wire which is straight, though the wire which is straight appears longer than the other one. Is this not the reason why you look smaller? |
| **Question:** | I am forty-five years old. Can I also follow your programme entitled, "Increase Your Height and Improve Your Posture?" |
| **Answer:** | If you are not suffering from any internal disease, you can undoubtedly follow our programme and achieve the desired results. You should not consider yourself to be too aged just at the age of forty-five. Be regular in your diet and habits and follow the directions given in our programme and see its magical results. |
| **Question:** | I am fourteen years old. The soles of my 'chappals' get rubbed off from inside. The outer corners of it do not get rubbed off. Why does it so happen? |
| **Answer:** | The position of your feet is defective and you walk with flat feet. Take a print of your feet on a thick paper. You will find that the style of your walking is not correct. (See Part II Step No. XVI. ) |
| **Question:** | I am fond of playing cricket and volleyball. Can I continue with these games while following your course on Increasing the Height? |

**Answer:**   No game is hurdle in our course. You can carry on with both of them. But you have to keep two things in mind: First that you should follow our course regularly. Do not give up any movement recommended for you. Second that you should not get yourself tired to such an extent that you do not get adequate rest, which is essential for increasing your height.

**Question:**   My son is thirteen years old. Can he also follow the course along with me?

**Answer:**   Why not? He can follow our course in the same way as you do. (As a matter of fact he can do it more quickly.) But you should bear in mind that the time for the various movements should be reduced to half for your son and that he should not be made to perform the more difficult and hard movements. It would be much better if you could get him medically examined first of all and seek the advice of a doctor before starting the course.

**Question:**   At what time should we perform the various exercises recommended in your course entitled "Increase Your Height and Improve Your Posture?"

**Answer:**   The best time to perform the various movements laid down in the course is that of the morning, when one has not taken anything. We have referred to this point while detailing the course. But if some one has no time in the morning, he can follow this course very conveniently three hours after his lunch.

**Question:**   There is Scoliosis in the backbone of my son. How does it happen? Is it also connected with one's stature?

**Answer:**   When children form the bad habit of leaning on one side while sitting, this unfortunate disease develops in the backbone. The defect

|  |  |
|---|---|
|  | should be removed by operation to be performed by a competent surgeon. When the patient becomes all right after operation, it is seen that his height increases by an inch or two. |
| **Question:** | I have crossed fifty years of age, but my stature has become shorter than before. How is it possible? |
| **Answer:** | As it is possible to increase your height in every age, so it is also possible for your stature to become short. If nourishing diet is not taken, the digestion is weak and there is lack of exercise, fresh air and sunshine, the skin dries up. The circulation of blood does not take place in the whole body. The different parts of the body of such a person shrink and become smaller. Thus not only the height of a person is reduced, but his weight also decreases. Sargeant Ya Kui, who wandered in the jungles during the Second World War, is a living example of this principle. Formerly his weight was 40 kilograms and height 150 cms. Due to absence of nourishing diet, his height was reduced by 20 cms., and the weight was also reduced by 8 kilograms. |
| **Question:** | I am very much short-statured. I do not feel confident that your course will help me to increase my height. What is your opinion? |
| **Answer:** | How can we say whether you will gain by our course or lose? When you do not have any faith in our course, you will follow it in a half-hearted manner. If you practise our course half-heartedly, the result will be so insignificant that you will not be able to perceive it. Our view is that if you begin any course with a sceptical attitude, you will end with despair. If you want to know about our faith in our course, we will point out that not only you, but hundreds and thousands of sceptics can fully gain by following |

|            | our course in the present, as they have done in the past. |
|------------|-----------|
| Question:  | What are the advantages of following your course? |
| Answer:    | Our course entitled "Increase Your Height and Improve Your Posture" is not a magic wand. We have never tried to please our admirers by making false promises. We have not even exaggerated the results. We have, throughout the course, laid emphasis on our understanding the peculiarities of human physiology and the effects produced on it by our diet, air, sunshine, rest, sleep, massage, exercise and the maintenance of right posture. Only after realizing the importance of these facts, you should talk about increasing your height. If you follow our course rightly, not only will your height increase, but your body will also become stout. You will become tall and healthy and will also come under the influence of Nature. |
| Question:  | "The height increases during night and shrinks during the day." How far is it correct? |
| Answer:    | It is a fact that the body is stretched at night and affords an opportunity and encouragement for one's stature to grow. When the man is asleep, the different parts of the vertebral system absorb the juices from the various sources in the body. Due to this process the different vertebrae get swollen up resulting in the increase of the length of the backbone. This is the main reason why the height of the person appears to have increased in the morning. When the man keeps himself busy during the day, the parts of the vertebral system shrink and the fluid present in them decreases. Consequently, the thickness of the various parts of the vertebral |

system is reduced and the height of the man is also reduced. Hence the height of a man is reduced in the evening as compared to his height in the morning by ½ cm. to ¾ cm. We, therefore, recommend nine to ten hours sleep for those persons who are desirous of increasing their height.

**Question:** I have given up your course mid-way. I have not followed your instructions fully. Even then people say that I look taller. My height has also increased. What is its reason?

**Answer:** If we reply to your question, we will have to indulge in self-praise. On the other hand we cannot believe that you have given up following our course. It appears that you are continuing with our course, but you are not aware of the same. *You must have imbibed the essentials of our course in your life such as, good diet, correct posture, following a daily routine, sleep and rest, and inhalation of fresh air.* These, too, are parts of our course, no doubt. But we are sorry to learn that that you have given up practising the movements recommended by us. If you would have continued practising these movements, you would have achieved so much success in increasing your height, which would have been beyond your imagination.

**Question:** You have referred to the neck of giraffe, while talking about the phenomenon of 'Increase in Height'. What do you want to derive from this?

**Answer:** Your question is very interesting. The tall neck of giraffe is the symbol of the success of one's will-power. It makes us recall that if we sincerely desire to increase our height, we can attain our goal. In the beginning, the giraffes had small necks. Once there was a famine. When they had eaten up all the leaves of trees which were nearby and easily accessible, they tried to raise their necks to eat the leaves of trees, which were at greater heights. Due to constant stretching of necks, they became taller.

The giraffe with tall necks gave birth to young ones having tall necks. Thus the necks of the giraffes became tall.

It is our firm conviction that if you have a strong will-power, you can attain more height than what is achieved naturally.

*Appendix*
## Useful Charts

## Dieting Chart Course No. 1
*Your diet to reduce your weight and fatness*

About 1200 calories

On getting up in the morning: Juice of lemon in cold or hot water. Tea without sugar.

**Breakfast**

| | |
|---|---|
| Toned Milk | 8 oz. (one glass) |
| Bread | 2 slices or |
| Dalia | 1 oz. |
| Corn Flakes | 1 oz. |

In between breakfast and lunch–
(If you take your lunch late)

Tea or coffee or fruit juice (without sugar)

**Lunch:**

| | |
|---|---|
| Flour | 3 small chapatis or |
| Rice | 2 oz. |
| Pulses | 1h oz. |
| Curd | 6 oz. or |
| Cheese | 2 oz. or |
| Meat, fish or chicken | 4 oz. |
| Vegetables | as much as you like. |

**Afternoon:**

Tea, or coffee or fruit juice
(without sugar)

| | |
|---|---|
| Salted Biscuits | 3 or |
| Cream Crackers | 2 |

**Dinner:**

    Similar to lunch

    Ghee or oil         2 teaspoonfuls
                          (for the whole day)

### Prohibited Food

1. Full cream milk, cream, butter, oil, ghee and fried articles.
2. Sugar, gur, bura, honey and sweets of all kinds.
3. Ovaltine, horlicks, coco etc.
4. Banana, mangoes ahd grapes.
5. Potato, gentleman's toe (arvi) and 'zaminkand'.
6. Coca cola and cold drinks.
7. Wine.

### Proposed diets

1. Vegetables, tomato, kheera, radish, lemon , vegetable or mutton soup, lassi, pickles,  chatni, zeera jal and amla.
2. Tea or coffee (without sugar).
3. Toned milk and articles made therefrom.

**Note:** If you like, you may take sacrine in place of sugar. If you suffer from high blood pressure along with fatness, you should not take salt, soda and sacrine.

# Dieting Chart Course No. 2

**Tested and tried diet schedule**
**Successful in removing fatness**
All India Institute of Medical Sciences,
Department of Dietary; New Delhi

*1,200 calories*                *Vegetarian/non-vegetarian*

**Breakfast:**

| | |
|---|---|
| Egg | 1 (not fried) |
| (or cheese) | 25 grams |
| Toned milk | 240 ml |
| Bread | 50 grams |
| Tea | |

97

**Lunch:**

| | |
|---|---|
| Pulses | 50 grams |
| Seasonal vegetables (cooked) | 375 grams |
| Curd | 100 grams |
| Chapati | 100 grams |
| Boiled rice | 100 grams |

**Dinner:**

| | |
|---|---|
| Meat, fish or chicken | 50 grams or |
| Cheese or grams | 25 grams |
| Cooked vegetables | 375 grams |
| Chapati | 100 grams |
| Rice | 100 grams |

OOO

# Major Minerals

| Mineral | Function | Rich Sources | Daily Recommendation |
|---|---|---|---|
| Calcium | Essential for healthy bones and teeth. | Found in abundance in milk and dairy products. Minor quantities can be found in dark green leafy vegetables, like spinach and watercress. | 700 mg for males and females. |
| Phosphorus | Promotes healthy cells, bones and teeth. | Milk, cheese, fish, meat and eggs. | 550 mg for males and females. |
| Magnesium | Helps the body use energy and muscles to function effectively. | Dark green leafy vegetables, like cabbage and broccoli. | 300 mg for males and females. |
| Sodium | Helps the body regulate its water content and nerves to function effectively. | As table salt, added to food for flavour. | 1,600 mg for males and females. |
| Potassium | Helps cells and body fluids function properly. | Most foods, apart from fats, oil and sugar. | 3,500 mg for males and females. |

# Trace Minerals

| Mineral | Function | Rich Sources | Daily Recommendation |
|---|---|---|---|
| Iron | Helps in formation of red blood cells; deficiency can cause anaemia. | Red meat, fortified cereals, bread, some fruits and vegetables. | 8.7 mg for males. 14.8 mg for females, more in case of heavy menstrual flow. |
| Zinc | Helps body reach sexual maturity and aids repair of damaged tissue. | Meat, fish, milk, cheese and eggs. | 9.5 mg for males. 7 mg for females. |
| Copper | Helps body use iron properly. | Green vegetables and fish. | 1.2 mg for males and females. |
| Selenium | Ensures healthy cells. | Meat, fish, cereals, eggs and cheese. | 75 µg for males. 60 µg for females. |
| Iodine | Helps make thyroid hormones, which control metabolic activity. | Seafood and dairy products. | 140 µg for males and females. |

# Vitamins

| Vitamin | Function | Overdose/ Toxicity | Rich Sources |
|---|---|---|---|
| Vitamin A | Prevents night blindness. Promotes healthy eye function. Keeps skin, hair, and nails healthy. Helps prevent bacterial infection. | Joint and bone pain, hair loss, skin changes, headaches, blurred vision, fatigue. | Green, yellow, or orange vegetables, cantaloupe, apricots, sweet potatoes, bananas, meats, poultry, fish, potatoes. |

# Vitamins

| Vitamin | Function | Overdose/ Toxicity | Rich Sources |
|---|---|---|---|
| Vitamin $B_6$ | Carbohydrates and protein metabolism. Helps form red blood cells. Promotes proper nerve function. | Nerve destruction. | Meats, poultry, fish, bananas, potatoes, broccoli, cereals and grains. |
| Vitamin $B_{12}$ | Promotes proper nerve function. | None known. | Meats, poultry, fish, milk, eggs. Vegetarians may need supplements. |
| Folic Acid | Helps form red blood cells. Builds genetic material. DNA and RNA synthesis. Helps form red blood cells. Important in growth and development. Helps prevent birth defects. | None known. | Orange and grapefruit juice, green leafy vegetables, dried beans, poultry. Supplements recommended for pregnancy. |
| Vitamin C | Promotes healing of cuts and wounds. Helps resist infection. Keeps gums healthy. Strengthens blood vessel walls. | Diarrhoea, kidney stones. | Citrus fruits (oranges, grapefruit), strawberries, cantaloupe, green or red peppers, broccoli. |
| Vitamin E | Helps form red blood cells, muscles, and other tissues. Antioxidant. | Muscle weakness, headaches, fatigue. | Seeds and nuts, seafood, eggs, oils. |

# Balanced Diets
*(The quantities are given in grams)*

| Food Item | Adult Man | | |
|---|---|---|---|
| | Sedentary | Moderate work | Heavy work |
| Cereals | 460 | 520 | 670 |
| Pulses | 40 | 50 | 60 |
| Leafy Vegetables | 40 | 40 | 40 |
| Other Vegetables | 60 | 70 | 80 |
| Roots and Tubers | 50 | 60 | 80 |
| Milk | 150 | 200 | 250 |
| Oil and Fat | 40 | 45 | 65 |
| Sugar or Jaggery | 30 | 35 | 55 |

# Balanced Diets
*(The quantities are given in grams)*

| Food Item | Adult Woman | | |
|---|---|---|---|
| | Sedentary | Moderate work | Heavy work |
| Cereals | 410 | 440 | 575 |
| Pulses | 40 | 45 | 50 |
| Leafy Vegetables | 100 | 100 | 50 |
| Other Vegetables | 40 | 40 | 100 |
| Roots and Tubers | 50 | 50 | 60 |
| Milk | 100 | 150 | 200 |
| Oil and Fat | 20 | 25 | 40 |
| Sugar or Jaggery | 20 | 20 | 40 |

## Balanced Diets
*(The quantities are given in grams)*

| Food Item | Children 1-3 years | Children 4-6 years | Boys 10-12 years | Girls 10-12 years |
|---|---|---|---|---|
| Cereals | 175 | 270 | 420 | 380 |
| Pulses | 35 | 35 | 45 | 45 |
| Leafy Vegetables | 40 | 50 | 50 | 50 |
| Other Vegetables | 20 | 30 | 50 | 50 |
| Roots and Tubers | 10 | 20 | 30 | 30 |
| Milk | 300 | 250 | 250 | 250 |
| Oil and Fat | 15 | 25 | 40 | 35 |
| Sugar or Jaggery | 30 | 40 | 45 | 45 |

Source: ICMR, *Recommended Dietary Intakes for Indians.*

## Recommended Calories for Indians

| Group | Particulars | Calories | Group | Particulars | Calories |
|---|---|---|---|---|---|
| Men | Sedentary work | 2,350 | Infants | 0–6 months | 118/kg |
| | Moderate work | 2,700 | | 6–12 months | 108/kg |
| | Heavy work | 3,200 | Children | 1–3 years | 1,125 |
| Women | Sedentary work | 1,800 | | 4–6 years | 1,600 |
| | Moderate work | 2,100 | | 7–9 years | 1,925 |
| | Heavy work | 2,450 | Boys | 10–12 years | 2,150 |
| | Pregnancy | +300 | | 13–15 years | 2,400 |
| | Lactation 0–6 months | +550 | | 16–18 years | 2,600 |
| | | | Girls | 10–12 years | 1,950 |
| | 6–12 months | +400 | | 13–15 years | 2,050 |
| | | | | 16–18 years | 2,150 |

Source: *National Institute of Nutrition, Hyderabad.*

## Standard Heights and Weights for Men and Women (Medium Frame) (For 25 years and above)

### MEN

| Height | | Weight (Kg.) |
|---|---|---|
| Cms. | Ft. | |
| 157 | 5' 2" | 56.3-60.3 |
| 160 | 5' 3" | 57.6-61.7 |
| 162 | 5' 4" | 58.9-63.5 |
| 165 | 5' 5" | 60.8-65.3 |
| 168 | 5' 6" | 62.2-66.7 |
| 170 | 5' 7" | 64.0-68.5 |
| 173 | 5' 8" | 65.8-70.8 |
| 175 | 5' 9" | 67.6-72.6 |
| 178 | 5' 10" | 69.4-74.4 |
| 180 | 5' 11" | 71.2-76.2 |
| 183 | 6' 0" | 73.0-78.5 |
| 185 | 6' 1" | 75.3-80.7 |
| 188 | 6' 2" | 77.6-83.5 |
| 190 | 6' 3" | 79.8-85.9 |

### WOMEN

| Height | | Weight (Kg.) |
|---|---|---|
| 152 | 5' 0" | 50.8-54.4 |
| 155 | 5' 1" | 51.7-55.3 |
| 157 | 5' 2" | 53.1-56.7 |
| 160 | 5' 3" | 54.4-58.1 |
| 162 | 5' 4" | 56.3-59.9 |
| 165 | 5' 5" | 57.6-61.2 |
| 168 | 5' 6" | 58.9-63.5 |
| 170 | 5' 7" | 60.8-65.3 |
| 173 | 5' 8" | 62.2-66.7 |
| 175 | 5' 9" | 64.0-68.5 |
| 178 | 5' 10" | 65.8-70.3 |
| 180 | 5' 11" | 67.1-71.7 |
| 183 | 6' 0" | 68.5-73.9 |

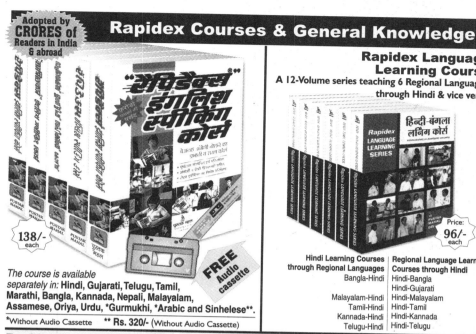
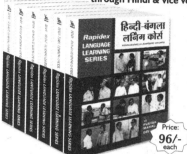
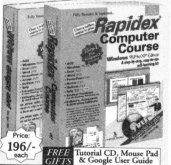
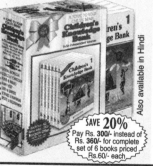
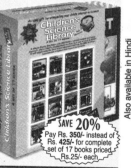
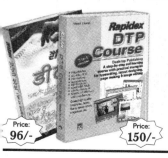
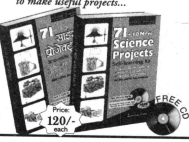
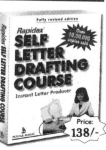
1

# Self-improvement

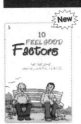

10 FEEL GOOD Factors

152 pp • Rs. 96/-

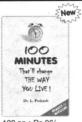

100 MINUTES That'll change THE WAY YOU LIVE!
Dr. L. Prakash

128 pp • Rs.96/-

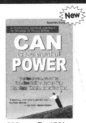

CAN is the word of POWER

292 pp • Rs.150/-

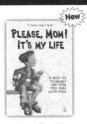

PLEASE, MOM! IT'S MY LIFE

112 pp • Rs. 80/-

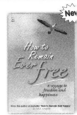

How to Remain Ever free

208 pp • Rs. 96/-

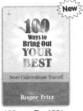

100 Ways to Bring Out YOUR BEST
Roger Fritz

168 pp • Rs. 120/-

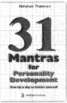

Abhishek Thakore's
31 Mantras for Personality Development

104 pp • Rs. 68/-

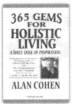

365 GEMS FOR HOLISTIC LIVING
A DAILY DOSE OF INSPIRATION
ALAN COHEN

376 pp • Rs. 120/-

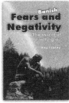

Banish Fears and Negativity

240 pp • Rs. 96/-

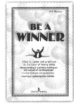

BE A WINNER

136 pp • Rs. 96/-

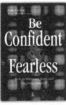

Be Confident Fearless

240 pp • Rs. 120/-

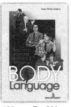

BODY Language

120 pp • Rs. 80/-
Also available in Hindi

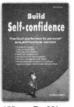

Build Self-confidence

155 pp • Rs. 80/-

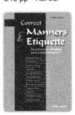

Correct Manners & Etiquette

156 pp • Rs. 80/-

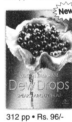

Dew Drops

312 pp • Rs. 96/-

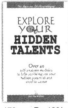

EXPLORE YOUR HIDDEN TALENTS

176 pp • Rs. 120/-

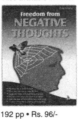

Freedom from NEGATIVE THOUGHTS

192 pp • Rs. 96/-

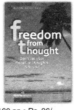

freedom from thought

160 pp • Rs. 96/-

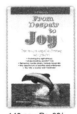

From Despair to Joy

140 pp • Rs. 80/-

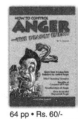

HOW TO CONTROL ANGER

64 pp • Rs. 60/-
Also available in Hind

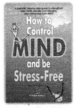

How to Control MIND and be Stress-Free

136 pp • Rs. 80/-
Also available in Hindi

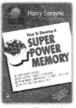

Harry Lorayne
How To Develop A SUPER POWER MEMORY

168 pp • Rs. 120/-

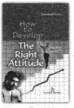

How to Develop The Right Attitude

96 pp • Rs. 68/-

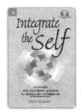

Integrate the Self

112 pp • Rs. 120/-
(with CD)

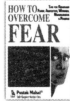

HOW TO OVERCOME FEAR

80 pp • Rs. 60/-
Also available in Hin

2

# Self-improvement

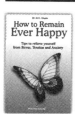

How to Remain Ever Happy
Tips to relieve yourself from Stress, Tension and Anxiety

160 pp • Rs. 80/-
Also in Hindi & Bangla

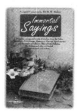

192 pp • Rs. 96/-

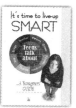

It's time to live-up SMART
Teens talk about
A Youngster's Guide

120 pp • Rs. 75/-
Earlier printed as
Teens to Twenties

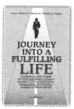

JOURNEY INTO A FULFILLING LIFE

176 pp • Rs. 68/-

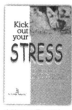

Kick out your STRESS

140 pp • Rs. 60/-

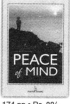

PEACE of MIND

174 pp • Rs. 88/-

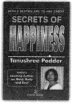

SECRETS OF HAPPINESS
Tanushree Podder

192 pp • Rs. 96/-

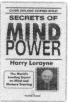

SECRETS OF MIND POWER
Harry Lorayne

184 pp • Rs. 96/-

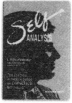

Self ANALYSIS

290 pp • Rs. 88/-

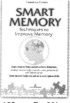

SMART MEMORY
Techniques to Improve Memory

138 pp • Rs. 80/-

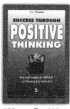

SUCCESS THROUGH POSITIVE THINKING

180 pp • Rs. 80/-

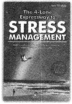

The 4-Lane Expressway to STRESS MANAGEMENT

112 pp • Rs. 95/-

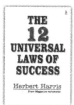

THE 12 UNIVERSAL LAWS OF SUCCESS
Herbert Harris

192 pp • Rs. 195/-

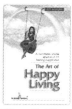

The Art of Happy Living

168 pp • Rs. 96/-

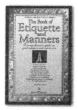

The Book of Etiquette and Manners

136 pp • Rs. 80/-

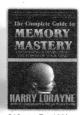

The Complete Guide to MEMORY MASTERY
HARRY LORAYNE

312 pp • Rs. 160/-

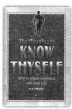

KNOW THYSELF

128 pp • Rs. 60/-

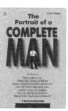

The Portrait of a COMPLETE MAN

176 pp • Rs. 96/-

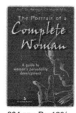

The Portrait of a Complete Woman

304 pp • Rs. 120/-

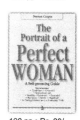

The Portrait of a Perfect WOMAN
A Self-grooming Guide

128 pp • Rs. 80/-

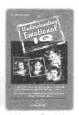

Understanding Emotional IQ

176 pp • Rs. 80/-

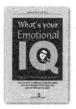

What's your Emotional IQ

176 pp • Rs. 68/-

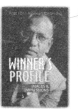

WINNER'S PROFILE

128 pp • Rs. 120/-

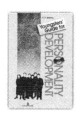

Youngsters' Guide for PERSONALITY DEVELOPMENT

120 pp • Rs. 80/-

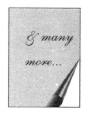

& many more...

3

# Career & Management

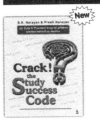

132 pp • Rs. 120/-

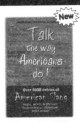

384 pp • Rs. 196/-

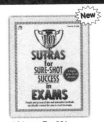

164 pp • Rs. 99/-

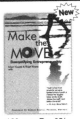

160 pp • Rs. 95/-

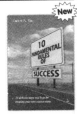

128 pp • Rs. 96/-

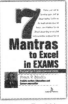

160 pp • Rs. 80/-
Also available in Hindi

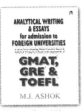

172 pp • Rs. 125/-

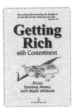

144 pp • Rs. 96/-

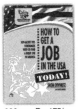

336 pp • Rs. 175/-

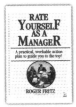

240 pp • Rs. 195/- (H

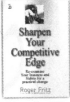

192 pp • Rs. 120/-

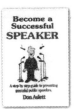

136 pp • Rs. 96/-

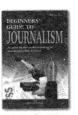

128 pp • Rs. 96/-

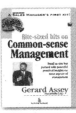

100 pp • Rs. 150/-

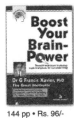

144 pp • Rs. 96/-

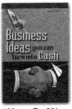

128 pp • Rs. 80/-

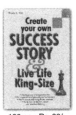

120 pp • Rs. 80/-

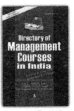

392 pp • Rs. 60/-

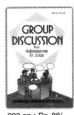

200 pp • Rs. 88/-

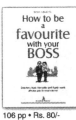

106 pp • Rs. 80/-

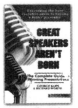

200 pp • Rs. 88/-

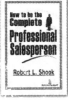

248 pp • Rs. 150/-

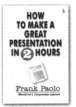

192 pp • Rs. 150/-

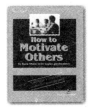

128 pp • Rs. 96/-

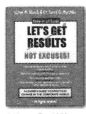

240 pp • Rs. 195/-

4

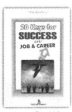

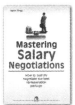

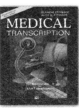

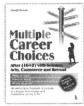

144 pp • Rs. 80/-   176 pp • Rs. 150/-   96 pp • Rs. 96/-   472 pp • Rs. 450/-   280 pp • Rs. 175/-

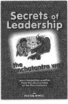

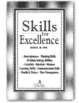

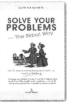

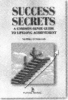

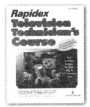

136 pp • Rs. 80/-   184 pp • Rs. 88/-   200 pp • Rs. 80/-   256 pp • Rs. 120/-   424 + Maps pp • Rs. 150/-

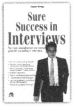

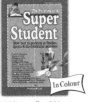

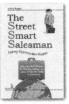

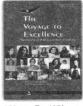

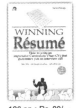

152 pp • Rs. 96/-   160/- pp • Rs. 80/-   208 pp • Rs. 88/-   280 pp • Rs. 195/-   136 pp • Rs. 80/-

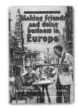

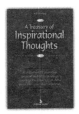

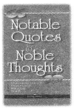

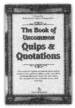

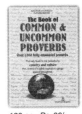

288 pp • Rs. 96/-   144 pp • Rs. 68/-   96 pp • Rs. 68/-   128 pp • Rs. 80/-   128 pp • Rs. 96/-

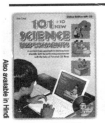

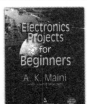

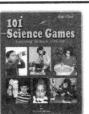

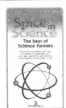

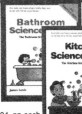

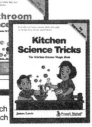

112 pp • Rs. 120/-
Coloured Ed. + FREE Tutorial CD

296 pp • Rs. 150/-

120 pp • Rs. 60/-
Also available in Hindi

144 pp • Rs. 60/-

104 pp each
Rs. 36/- each

# Health, Yogasana & Body Fitness

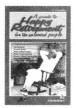
128 pp • Rs. 60/-

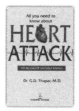
152 pp • Rs. 96/-

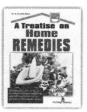
224 pp • Rs. 120/-

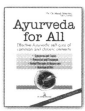
224 pp • Rs. 150/-

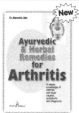
192 pp • Rs. 96/-

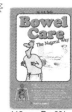
112 pp • Rs. 60/-

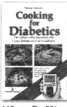
115 pp • Rs. 80/-

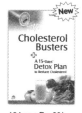
104 pp • Rs. 60/-

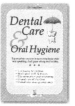
136 pp • Rs. 96/-

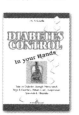
120 pp • Rs. 88/-

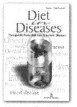
104 pp • Rs. 69/-

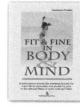
232 pp • Rs. 90/-

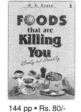
144 pp • Rs. 80/-

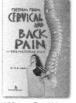
128 pp • Rs. 68/-

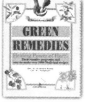
243 pp • Rs. 160/-

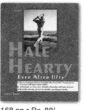
168 pp • Rs. 88/-

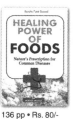
136 pp • Rs. 80/-

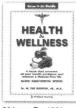
304 pp • Rs. 120/-

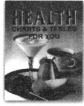
144 pp • Rs. 96/-

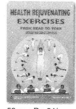
52 pp • Rs. 24/-

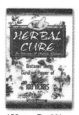
152 pp • Rs. 88/-

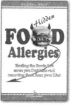
126 pp • Rs. 80/-

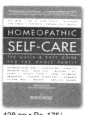
428 pp • Rs. 175/-

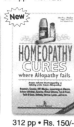
312 pp • Rs. 150/-

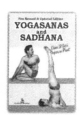
176 pp • Rs. 60/-

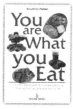
180 pp • Rs. 80/-

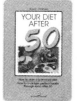
150 pp • Rs. 68/-

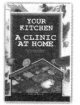
128 pp • Rs. 68/-

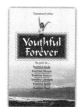
242 pp • Rs. 80/-

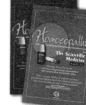
140 pp • Rs. 96/- (Vol.
224 pp • Rs. 135/- (Vol.

Health, Yogasana & Body Fitness

# Health, Yogasana & Body Fitness

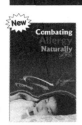
120 pp • Rs. 88/-

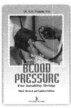
128 pp • Rs. 96/-

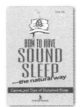
136 pp • Rs. 68/-

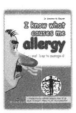
96 pp • Rs. 40/-

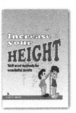
112 pp • Rs. 60/-
Also in Hindi & Bangla

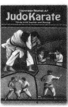
128 pp • Rs. 48/-
Also in Hindi & Bangla

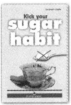
96 pp • Rs. 48/-

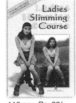
112 pp • Rs. 60/-
(Also available in Hindi)

120 pp • Rs. 80/-

176 pp • Rs. 96/-

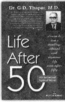
192 pp • Rs. 120/-

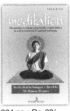
224 pp • Rs. 88/-

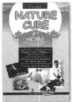
232 pp • Rs. 80/-
Also available in Hindi

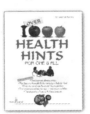
168 pp • Rs. 80/-

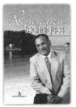
272 pp • Rs. 195/-

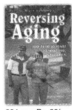
224 pp • Rs. 80/-

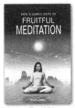
96 pp • Rs. 80/-

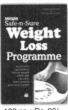
132 pp • Rs. 96/-

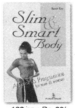
128 pp • Rs. 80/-

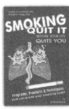
192 pp • Rs. 68/-

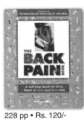
228 pp • Rs. 120/-

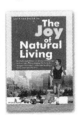
152 pp • Rs. 80/-

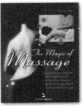
176 pp • Rs. 110/-

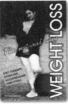
128 pp • Rs. 68/-

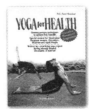
184 pp • Rs. 120/-

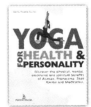
124 pp • Rs. 96/-

# Alternative Therapies

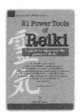
136 pp • Rs. 60/-

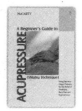
64 pp • Rs. 48/-

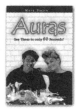
144 pp • Rs. 88/-

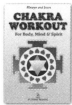
240 pp • Rs. 88/-

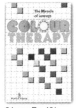
84 pp • Rs. 48/-

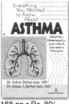
168 pp • Rs. 80/-

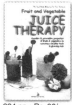
224 pp • Rs. 96/-

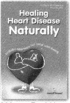
200 pp • Rs. 96/-

180 pp • Rs. 68/-

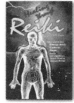
104 pp • Rs. 60/-

120 pp • Rs. 60/-

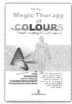
128 pp • Rs. 68/-

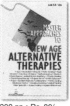
200 pp • Rs. 80/-

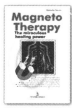
128 pp • Rs. 80/-

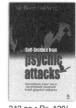
242 pp • Rs. 120/-

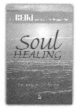
280 pp • Rs. 96/-

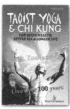
304 pp • Rs. 120/-

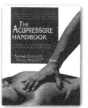
264 pp • Rs. 150/-

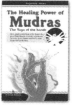
112 pp • Rs. 80/-

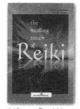
112 pp • Rs. 68/-

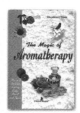
264 pp • Rs. 108/-

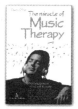
144 pp • Rs. 80/-

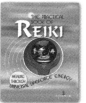
168 pp • Rs. 96/-

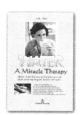
112 pp • Rs. 68/-

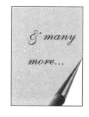
& many more...

# Palmistry, Hypnotism, Astrology & Numerology

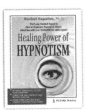
264 pp • Rs. 150/-

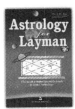
184 pp • Rs. 80/-

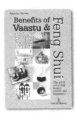
144 pp • Rs. 88/-

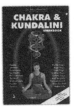
264 pp • Rs. 110/-

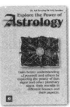
200 pp • Rs. 96/-

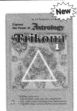
208 pp • Rs. 125/-

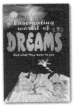
144 pp • Rs. 60/-

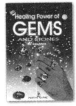
136 pp • Rs. 80/-

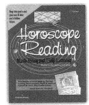
248 pp • Rs. 135/-

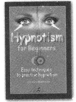
160 pp • Rs. 75/-

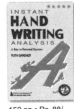
152 pp • Rs. 88/-

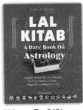
336 pp • Rs. 240/-
Hardbound

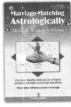
142 pp • Rs. 80/-

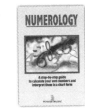
272 pp • Rs. 96/-

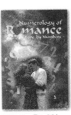
222 pp • Rs. 80/-

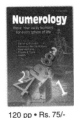
120 pp • Rs. 75/-

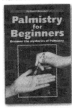
282 pp • Rs. 88/-

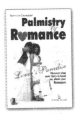
180 pp • Rs. 80/-

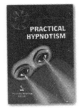
236 pp • Rs. 75/-
Also available in Hindi

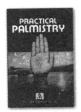
365 pp • Rs. 80/-
Also available in Hindi

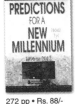
272 pp • Rs. 88/-

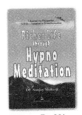
107 pp • Rs. 80/-

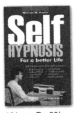
184 pp • Rs. 96/-

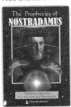
160 pp • Rs. 60/-
Also available in Hindi

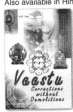
92 pp • Rs. 72/-

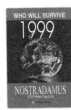
304 pp • Rs. 75/-

# Dictionaries, Encyclopedias, World Famous etc.

128 pp • Rs. 68/-

220 pp • Rs. 80/-

231 pp • Rs. 120/-

196 pp • Rs. 60/-

58 pp • Rs. 72/-

48 pp • Rs. 48/-

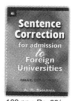
168 pp • Rs. 60/-

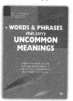
136 pp • Rs. 50/-

136 pp • Rs. 60/-

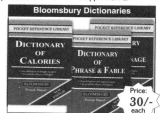
**Bloomsbury Dictionaries**
Price: 30/- each

--- pp • Rs. 108/-

520 pp • Rs. 380/-

344 pp • Rs. 120/-

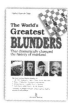
128 pp • Rs. 68/-

128 pp • Rs. 60/-

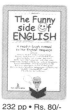
232 pp • Rs. 80/-

## World Famous

Rs.60/- each
Also in Hindi

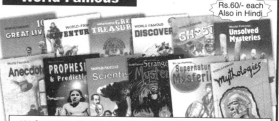

101 Great Lives (3 vols.) • Adventures • Great Treasures • Discoveries • Ghosts • Anecdotes • Unsolved Mysteries • Prophesies & Predictions • Scientists • Strange Mysteries • Supernatural Mysteries • Mythologies

**Famous Indians of 20th Century**
224 pp • Rs. **120/-**

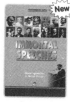
**Immortal Speeches**
136 pp • Rs. **80/-**

**J. Krishnamurty and Problems of Human Life**
168 pp • Rs. **80/-**

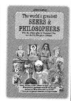
**The World's Greatest Seers & Philosophers**
224 pp • Rs. **120/-**

### Furniture Catalogue, Gates, Grills, Windows, Railings...

New Furniture Catalogue

200 pp • Rs. 150/-

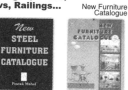
120 pp • Rs. 195/-
256 pp • Rs. 150/-

56 pp • Rs. 72/-

136 pp • Rs. 60/-

88 pp • Rs. 60/-

88 pp • Rs. 60/-

88 pp • Rs. 60/-

136 pp • Rs. 90/-

# Computer, Quiz Books / Love, Romance & Sex

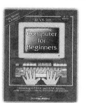

192 pp • Rs. 80/-

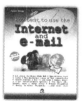

136 pp • Rs. 99/-

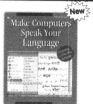

New

208 pp • Rs. 175/-

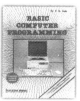

264 pp • Rs. 80/-

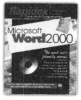

448 pp • Rs. 175/-

520 pp • Rs. 195/-

## Rapidex Straight to the Point Series

## Rapidex Condensed Users Guides

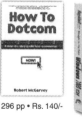

296 pp • Rs. 140/-

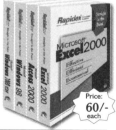

Price: 60/- each

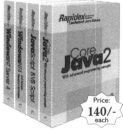

Price: 140/- each

## LOVE, ROMANCE & SEX

144 pp • Rs. 60/-

128 pp • Rs. 80/-

64 pp • Rs. 30/-

120 pp • Rs. 60/-

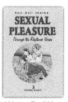

160 pp • Rs. 80/-

116 pp • Rs. 60/-

120 pp • Rs. 60/-

208 pp • Rs. 160/-

## QUIZ BOOKS

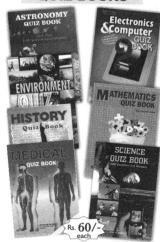

Rs. 60/- each

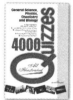

240 pp • Rs. 88/-

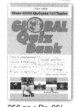

256 pp • Rs. 96/-

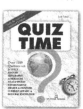

208 pp • Rs. 96/-
Also available in Bangla

## Other Computer Books

| | |
|---|---|
| The Wap Book | 99/- |
| The Java Book | 195/- |
| Dreamweaver 3 | 195/- |
| Low-cost Web Site | 225/- |
| Internet Marketing & Promotions | 225/- |
| Microsoft FrontPage 8 | 90/- |
| Microsoft Outlook 2000 | 125/- |
| E-Strategy | 120/- |

■ 11

# Religion & Parenting

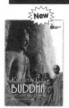
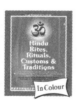
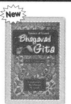

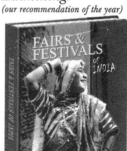
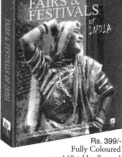

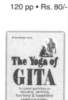

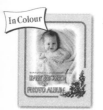
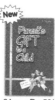
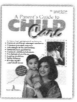
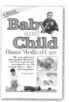

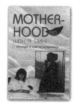

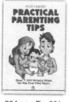

# Cookery, Women Orientation, Beauty

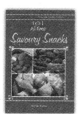
102 pp • Rs. 60/-

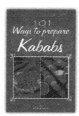
136 pp • Rs. 80/-

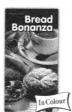
152 pp • Rs. 125/-

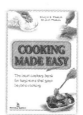
104 pp • Rs. 60/-

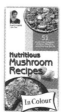
96 pp • Rs. 96/-

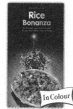
144 pp • Rs. 125/-

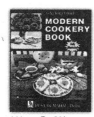
144 pp • Rs. 80/-
Also in Hindi

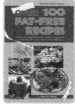
120 pp • Rs. 80/-

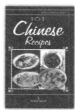
112 pp • Rs. 60/-

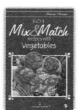
144 pp • Rs. 80/-

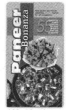
168+16 colour pp
Rs. 80/-

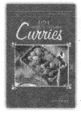
140 pp • Rs. 60/-

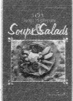
86 pp • Rs. 80/-

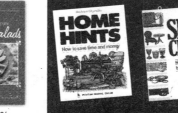
32 pp each • Rs. 40/- each

& many more...

192 pp • Rs. 120/-

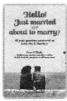
144 pp • Rs. 80/-

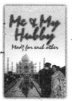
248 pp • Rs. 96/-

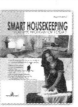
296 pp • Rs. 150/-

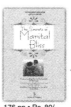
176 pp • Rs. 80/-

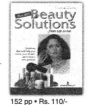
152 pp • Rs. 110/-

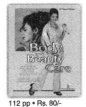
112 pp • Rs. 80/-

128 pp • Rs. 80/-
Also available in Hindi

128 pp • Rs. 80/-

144 pp • Rs. 75/-
Also available in Hindi

124 pp • Rs. 60/-

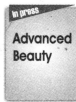

13

# Humour, Fun, Facts, Magic & Hobbies

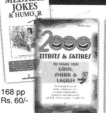
168 pp
Rs. 60/-

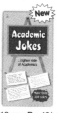
176 pp • Rs. 68/-

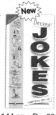
112 pp • Rs. 48/-

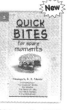
144 pp • Rs. 60/-

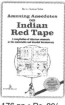
224 pp • Rs. 120/-

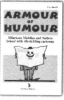
176 pp • Rs. 80/-

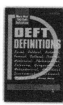
128 pp • Rs. 40/-

120 pp • Rs. 48/-

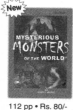
112 pp • Rs. 80/-

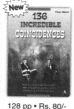
128 pp • Rs. 80/-

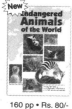
160 pp • Rs. 80/-

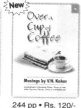
244 pp • Rs. 120/-

128 pp • Rs. 60/-

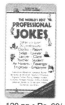
120 pp • Rs. 60/-

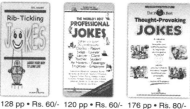
176 pp • Rs. 80/-

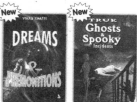
152 pp • Rs. 80/-

136 pp • Rs. 80/-

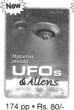
174 pp • Rs. 80/-

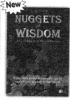
112 pp • Rs. 80/-

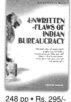
248 pp • Rs. 295/-
(Hardbound)

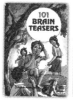
152 pp • Rs. 68/-
also available in Hindi

112 pp • Rs. 96/-

115 pp • Rs. 48/-
also available in Hindi

104 pp • Rs. 48/-
also in Hindi,
Bangla, Kannada &
Assamese

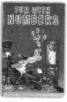
115 pp • Rs. 48/-
also in Hindi

112 pp • Rs. 48/-
also in Hindi

112 pp • Rs.48/-
also in Hindi,
Kannada and Marathi

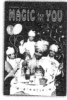
124 pp • Rs. 48/-
also in Hindi

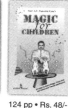
124 pp • Rs. 48/-
also in Hindi

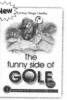
96 pp • Rs. 100/-

104 pp • Rs. 60/-

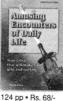
124 pp • Rs. 68/-

180 pp • Rs. 68/-

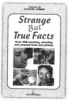
184 pp • Rs. 80/-

120 pp • Rs. 60/-
Also available in Hindi

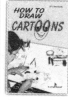
124 pp • Rs. 68/-
Also available in Hindi